TAKE CHARGE OF YOUR DIABETES

TAKE CHARGE
OF YOUR DIABETES

A Revolutionary Plan for
Treating Your Diabetes and
Preventing Its Complications

SARFRAZ ZAIDI, M.D.

WITH
Georgie Huntington Zaidi

Da Capo
LIFE
LONG
A Member of the Perseus Books Group
New York

Printed in the United States of America.

Da Capo Press is a member of the Perseus Books Group.

Text design by BackStory Design
Set in 11.5 Sabon

First printing, May 2007

Visit us on the World Wide Web at www.perseusbooksgroup.com

A CIP record for this book is available from the Library of Congress.
ISBN-13: 978-0-7382-1099-5
ISBN-10: 0-7382-1099-4

Da Capo Press books are available at special discounts for bulk purchases in the U.S. by corporations, institutions, and other organizations. For more information, please contact the Special Markets Department at the Perseus Books Group, 2300 Chestnut St., Philadelphia, PA 19103, or e-mail special.markets@perseusbooks.com.

1 2 3 4 5 6 7 8 9

I dedicate this book to my patients,
who have been my best teachers

CONTENTS

PART III

Preventing, Stopping, and Even Reversing Complications of Diabetes

TAKE CHARGE OF YOUR DIABETES

Introduction

George, a Caucasian male, came to see me for his diabetes, after undergoing three angioplasties in two years. Despite following his doctor's advice—adhering to a conventional antidiabetic regimen of a special diet, more exercise, and insulin injections—he developed severe coronary artery disease. He was obviously quite demoralized. It shouldn't have to be this way.

In the last fifteen years, there has been a tremendous amount of research in the field of diabetes, and the resulting treatment changes are revolutionary. Unfortunately, most doctors have not embraced these new scientific developments. They continue to treat diabetes with an outdated, conventional approach that merely focuses on lowering blood glucose but does not treat the underlying root cause of diabetes. It's like trying to halt the growth of a poisonous tree by trimming its branches. Meanwhile, the roots continue to grow stronger.

Using new scientific research and developments, I developed a revolutionary approach to treating diabetes. With my new treatment strategy, most diabetic patients can avoid insulin injections and do well with new oral medications. They can truly prevent deadly complications of diabetes! Those who have already developed complications, like George, can prevent further damage.

Most people develop diabetes due to a complex disease process in their body known as insulin resistance. It takes many years of insulin resistance before you become diabetic. During this time, insulin resistance causes many other changes in your body that are quite harmful. For example, insulin resistance increases serum triglycerides (the fat in blood), lowers HDL cholesterol (the good cholesterol), and changes LDL cholesterol (the bad cholesterol) from Type A (less dangerous) to Type B (more dangerous). In addition, insulin resistance increases blood pressure, makes it easier for blood to clot, and impairs our body's natural ability to break down blood clots. All of these abnormalities set the stage for a heart attack and/or stroke.

When I first saw George, his diabetes was out of control despite insulin shots. He was on the usual, conventional treatment for diabetes. For years, he took glyburide, an oral medication, which initially controlled his blood glucose. Predictably, after a few years, his blood glucose started escalating, and glyburide was of no help.

Glyburide is an old drug and belongs to the class of drugs known as sulfonylurea drugs. Other drugs in this class include glipizide, glimepiride, and chlorpropamide. Before 1994, these were the only oral drugs available in the U.S. for the treatment of Type 2 diabetes. These sulfonylurea drugs act by stimulating the pancreas to produce more insulin, but they do not treat insulin resistance. This treatment is like flogging a tired horse. Eventually the horse slows down, stumbles, and drops dead.

George's exhausted pancreas, like a tired horse, could not produce enough insulin despite stimulation from sulfonylurea drugs. Eventually, he had to go on insulin shots to control his diabetes. However, once again, this was an ineffective strategy. The reason? Like sulfonylurea drugs, insulin shots do not treat insulin resistance. Eventually, most diabetic patients using insulin shots, like

George, develop coronary heart disease requiring angioplasties or even heart bypass surgery. They are also at a high risk for a stroke and leg amputation.

Ten years ago, I realized that to effectively treat Type 2 diabetics, insulin resistance must be treated first and foremost. I developed a new, revolutionary, and still cutting-edge strategy that focuses on treating insulin resistance instead of merely chasing blood sugar levels. Once insulin resistance is treated, the burden of excessive insulin production on the pancreas is gone. Relieved of the stress of overproducing insulin, the pancreas begins to work efficiently again. As a result, patients achieve long-lasting control of blood sugars without stressing the pancreas. They do not have to resort to insulin injections. Many of those who are already on insulin shots can gradually be weaned off.

My new treatment plan, outlined in this book, not only controls diabetes but also reduces serum triglycerides, increases HDL (good) cholesterol, changes LDL cholesterol from Type B (more dangerous) to Type A (less dangerous), and re-establishes the body's ability to break clots. It accomplishes these major goals by effectively treating insulin resistance—the root cause of these medical disorders. In this way, my new treatment strategy significantly reduces the risk for heart attack, stroke, leg amputation, dementia, kidney disease, and other complications of diabetes. Those who already have gone through a coronary angioplasty can stop the vicious cycle of repeated angioplasties. Those who have suffered a stroke can prevent future episodes. Those with memory loss and dementia can prevent further deterioration. Those who have developed an early stage of kidney disease can prevent further progression and avoid ending up on kidney dialysis. Patients with diabetes can now prevent leg amputation and blindness.

This certainly has been my clinical experience as the director of the Jamila Diabetes & Endocrine Medical Center. By using this new treatment strategy, the majority of my diabetic patients do not need to resort to insulin shots to control their diabetes. Most of those patients who are already on insulin injections gradually come off insulin. Most of my diabetic patients have *not* required coronary angioplasties, heart bypass surgery, or kidney dialysis. Patients with previous strokes have *not* suffered any further episodes. There have been *no* leg amputations or loss of eyesight in many years.

George has benefited from this new treatment plan. Once I started treating his insulin resistance, his diabetes came under much better control. Gradually, I took him off insulin. I think it's fair to say that he was quite thrilled that he no longer had to endure insulin injections. More impressively, as of this writing, he hasn't had a single coronary angioplasty in eight years.

In this book you will learn about my revolutionary treatment strategy for diabetic patients. I will explain insulin resistance and how it leads to diabetes and its complications. You will understand how to cut the poisonous tree of diabetes at its roots rather than merely trimming its branches.

Insulin resistance is caused by five factors. Therefore, my treatment plan consists of five corresponding pillars: an easy-to-follow diet, a sensible exercise program, a unique stress management strategy, an unbiased review of vitamins and herbs, and a detailed discussion about drugs.

Throughout the explanation of this five-pillar treatment plan, you'll find real-life case studies from my practice to emphasize and explain my points. It's my hope that you'll start to understand the reality of what is happening in your body and how you can turn things around. My treatment starts to work right away. In a couple of months, you will have made a U-turn and be on a completely different road. Indeed, by the end of this book, you will know how to take charge of your diabetes!

PART ONE

UNDERSTANDING AND DIAGNOSING DIABETES

CHAPTER 1

What Is Diabetes?

To truly understand my new treatment strategy, you first need to understand what is going on in your body. Those of you who think you already know what diabetes is, think again. In fact, forget everything you've already learned! Much of what you've learned is likely filled with misinformation and errors. Many magazine articles are full of incorrect information. Even some doctors may confuse their patients with poor explanations.

When you build a house, you start with a strong foundation. Similarly, if you want to take charge of your diabetes, you need to start with a strong foundation in your knowledge of diabetes and how it develops and affects your body. So wipe out what you think you know about diabetes and let's start over and get the facts straight.

Most people mistakenly think that diabetes is simply a matter of elevated blood glucose. Take care of high blood glucose and you will be fine. Not true! In the majority of patients, diabetes is one of the manifestations of a seriously harmful disease process in the body called insulin resistance. Simply put, insulin resistance means your own insulin—a hormone naturally produced by the pancreas—becomes less effective in doing its job. In response to this insulin resistance, the pancreas produces more and more insulin so that blood glucose levels remain normal. Eventually the pancreas is unable to continue churning out these huge amounts of insulin, and blood glucose levels start to rise.

Usually, it takes several years before your blood glucose rises to a level that is diagnostic for diabetes. But during this time, the process of insulin resistance is taking a toll on your body by narrowing your blood vessels, depositing fat into your liver, and contributing to the growth of cancer in your body. That is why these patients often experience a heart attack or stroke before they are diagnosed with diabetes.

Diabetes is only one of the manifestations of insulin resistance in the majority of diabetic patients. Other manifestations include high blood pressure, cholesterol disorder, heart disease, stroke, dementia, fatty liver, and a high risk for cancer. Understanding this distinction is the first step toward taking charge of your condition. Before moving ahead to treatment options, however, it's important to understand the different kinds of diabetes.

Types of Diabetes

Basically, there are three types of diabetes mellitus: Type 1, Type 2, and gestational.

Type 1 Diabetes

Only a minority (about 5%) of diabetic patients are Type 1. In this disease, there is a complete destruction of insulin producing cells (called beta cells) in the pancreas by the person's own immune system. Consequently, insulin, an essential chemical produced by the pancreas, stops being produced.

One of the main functions of insulin is to drive glucose from the blood into the cells, especially muscle cells, where it is used as a fuel to produce energy. Think of the cell as a small room and the blood vessel as a hallway outside of the room. Glucose is a delivery person, running through the hallway trying to enter the room, but the door is closed. Insulin works as the doorman, opening the door for glucose to enter.

When there is a complete lack of insulin (the doorman is gone), as happens with Type 1 diabetes, the door to the cell remains closed, which causes a rapid buildup of glucose in the blood. A markedly high level of glucose in the blood leads to the sudden onset of excessive thirst, frequent urination, weight loss, and fatigue. Patients with Type 1 diabetes have to take insulin on a regular basis. If they stop taking insulin, they can rapidly lapse into a coma and die if treatment is not instituted in time.

Type 2 Diabetes

The majority (about 95%) of diabetic patients are Type 2. In contrast to Type 1 diabetics, most Type 2 diabetics do not need insulin shots to manage their diabetes. In Type 2 diabetes, the body is able to produce insulin, but there is resistance to its action. This is known as insulin resistance.

Remember, insulin works as a doorman. It must open the door for glucose to enter a cell. In individuals prone to develop Type 2 diabetes, the door hinges of the cell are rusty. Consequently, insulin cannot easily open the door. Now, instead of one doorman, you need three or four doormen to pry the door open. This is called insulin resistance.

In response to insulin resistance, the pancreas produces more and more insulin. This keeps your blood sugar in the normal range for a long time. But if insulin resistance is not treated, the pancreas eventually becomes exhausted and insulin production starts to drop. At this stage, your blood glucose levels start to rise, and you gradually develop prediabetes and then diabetes.

The ability of the pancreas to produce insulin varies from person to person. Some people have a limited ability to produce insulin and they develop diabetes only after a few years of insulin resistance. Others have a tremendous reserve for insulin production and do not develop diabetes for many years despite ongoing insulin resistance.

Gestational Diabetes

Gestational diabetes refers to the development of diabetes during pregnancy. After a pregnancy ends, most women with gestational diabetes return to "normal" blood glucose ranges. However, within ten years, more than 50% of women with gestational diabetes will develop Type 2 diabetes and, therefore, should be closely monitored for the development of diabetes.

Symptoms of Diabetes

You've been putting it off, but finally you go to your doctor's office for your annual checkup. Two days later the doctor calls you with results from your lab test and, unfortunately, it's bad news. You have diabetes! "But, but, I feel fine!" you stammer. "It must be a mistake. I don't have frequent urination. No one in my family had diabetes." But you are actually one of the lucky ones. Many people don't realize they have diabetes until they're in the hospital having a heart attack or stroke.

Only a few people have classic symptoms like frequent urination and excessive thirst. Many have nonspecific symptoms such as fatigue or tingling in the toes. Sometimes, people just assume that they're just getting old and tired.

Not knowing you have diabetes is like having mold in your house without knowing it's what is causing all your awful allergies. Once you discover that mold is the root of your problem, you can do something about it. In the same way, it's better to know you have diabetes. Then you can take control and do something about it!

Diabetes patients may ultimately develop any of the following symptoms:

- Tingling, numbness, a burning sensation or pain in toes, fingers, or both
- Chest pain/heart attack
- Stroke
- Memory loss
- Impotence
- Blurry vision
- Excessive thirst
- Frequent urination
- Drowsiness, coma
- Susceptibility to and difficulty in clearing up infections

Excessive thirst and urination, blurry vision, and drowsiness are usually symptoms of severe diabetes.

Type 1 diabetics usually have more dramatic symptoms such as:

- Weight loss
- Excessive thirst

- Frequent urination, especially waking up several times a night to urinate
- A life-threatening condition known as diabetic ketoacidosis (DKA). In this condition, a patient may experience nausea, vomiting, abdominal pain, mental confusion, drowsiness, and can even lapse into a coma. These patients usually have a fruity smell on their breath.

Patients with DKA are usually Type 1 diabetics, although it rarely can occur in Type 2 diabetics, as well.

Categorizing Your Diabetes

An endocrinologist, the diabetes expert, can diagnose whether you have Type 1 or Type 2 diabetes based upon clinical information. Unfortunately, a physician who is not a diabetes specialist may incorrectly categorize the kind of diabetes you have.

You Are Probably a Type 2 Diabetic If:

- You are not on insulin
- You are on insulin but in the past you were successfully treated with diabetic pills for several years before you were placed on insulin
- You are on relatively large doses of insulin (usually more than 40 units/day)
- You are obese
- You have high triglycerides (more than 150 mg/dl)
- You have low HDL cholesterol (less than 50mg/dl in females and less than 40 mg/dl in males)

Age Has No Bearing on Your Type of Diabetes

In the past, we erroneously used to classify Type 1 diabetes as "Juvenile Onset Diabetes" and Type 2 diabetes as "Adult Onset" or "Maturity Onset." But then we realized that many young people were actually not Type 1 but Type 2. As a matter of fact, Type 2 diabetes among teenagers is increasing at an alarming rate, thanks to our culture of fast food and a sedentary lifestyle.

Type 1 diabetes can rarely develop in adults. Therefore, now we use the terms Type 1 or Type 2 and don't use the previous, age-related categories. Sadly, I see some physicians still using the old terms. Presuming someone has Type 1 diabetes based upon their young age can be very misleading.

- You have high blood pressure (more than 130/85 mm Hg)
- You have a family history of diabetes, high blood pressure, heart disease, stroke, or high cholesterol

You Are Probably a Type 1 Diabetic If:

- You have been on insulin ever since the diagnosis of your diabetes or shortly thereafter (although sometimes your physician may erroneously place you on insulin even though you are a Type 2 diabetic)
- You are on relatively small doses of insulin (usually less than 40 units/day)
- You are thin
- You do not have a family history of diabetes
- You do not have high triglycerides and low HDL cholesterol
- You do not have high blood pressure

Blood Testing to Categorize the Type of Diabetes

There is a special blood test that can help categorize whether a person is Type 1 or Type 2. This blood test is known as C-peptide, which is a hormone produced by the pancreas in conjunction with insulin.

The blood test for C-peptide should be done one hour after a meal.

Almost all Type 2 diabetic patients have some production of insulin and C-peptide. Actually, many Type 2 diabetics have excessive production of insulin and an elevated level of C-peptide. In contrast, most Type 1 diabetics have no insulin production and, therefore, no C-peptide in their blood.

Rarely, and only in small quantities, is C-peptide detectable in the early stages of Type 1 diabetes. In these difficult cases, further blood testing, such as anti-islet cell antibodies or anti-GAD antibodies, can be carried out. These antibodies are present in most patients with Type 1 diabetes.

Let me share a real case from my medical practice to demonstrate how I use clinical information and blood tests to categorize a patient's diabetes type. At the young age of thirty, David, a Caucasian male, was diagnosed with Type 1 diabetes and placed on insulin. Demoralized and frustrated, he took several injections of insulin a day, but his blood glucose remained high, in the 200 mg/dl range most of the time. Each visit to his doctor produced the same response: "Increase your insulin dose, David." David didn't understand why his diabetes was so out of control despite all that insulin he was injecting. Over six years, he saw four different physicians, attended several diabetes education sessions, and thought he knew everything about diabetes. Finally, he came to see me.

When I first saw David, I had a strong clinical impression that he was not a Type 1, but in fact, a Type 2 diabetic. Why? Because David was obese, especially around his waistline. He had a family history of Type 2 diabetes, and he was on large doses of insulin, about 140 units/day. When I first told him that he was probably a Type 2 diabetic, he was shocked. Later, he confessed that he did not initially believe me. "How could all the other doctors treating me in the last six years be wrong?"

So, I ordered a C-peptide for David. It turned out to be high at 6.0 ng/ml (normal range is 0.8–3.1). It confirmed my clinical impression that David indeed was a Type 2 diabetic. I took him off insulin and started him on my new approach to treating Type 2 diabetes. Within a month, his blood glucose values dropped from the 200–300 mg/dl range to about the 100–130 mg/dl range. Four months later, his hemoglobin A1c (a measure of overall blood glucose control in a three-month period) dropped from 7.8% to 6.6%. David was thrilled—not only was he able to stop insulin shots, but his diabetes was under control for the first time since he had been diagnosed.

You Can Be Either Type 1 or Type 2, but Never Both

Some people mistakenly think they have Type 1 as well as Type 2 diabetes. Others think that they were originally Type 2 and later progressed to Type 1. To my surprise, even some physicians have these misconceptions.

Type 1 and Type 2 diabetes are two different disease processes. You have one or the other. You do not progress from one to the other. There is no crossover.

In Type 1 diabetes, there is complete destruction of insulin producing cells in the pancreas and, consequently, your body no longer produces insulin. You must take insulin on a regular basis to survive.

In Type 2 diabetes, the body is able to produce insulin, but there is resistance to the action of insulin. It is a completely different disease from Type 1 diabetes.

Unfortunately, many Type 2 diabetics are treated according to the "usual, conventional" treatment strategy with drugs that stimulate the pancreas to produce more and more insulin while nothing is done to reduce insulin resistance. The pancreas eventually exhausts and dries out—unable to produce enough insulin to meet the huge demands due to insulin resistance. At that point, patients are placed on insulin injections to control their blood glucose. Some patients (and surprisingly some physicians) erroneously think that their diabetes converted from Type 2 to Type 1 and they will have to stay on insulin for the rest of their life.

In fact, if Type 2 diabetics are treated with my new approach, they do not develop pancreatic exhaustion, and they do not have to go on insulin. Even those Type 2 diabetics who are already on insulin injections can gradually come off insulin by using my new approach that rejuvenates the pancreas. My recommended protocol is discussed in detail in Part II.

If you are Type 2, then your physician, in consultation with an endocrinologist, can attempt to gradually take you off insulin. But take note: you must never stop insulin on your own!

If you are a Type 1 diabetic, you still may develop insulin resistance as you grow older and gain excessive weight. You will require larger doses of insulin to control your blood glucose and have other manifestations of insulin resistance as discussed in detail in chapter 2.

CHAPTER 2

What Causes Diabetes?

Before we discuss the treatment of diabetes, you must fully understand what caused your diabetes. Only then can you truly understand the distinctions and advantages of my approach to treatment.

More than 95% of diabetics are Type 2. The root cause for Type 2 diabetes is a disease process in your body known as insulin resistance. Therefore, insulin resistance is the underlying problem for the great majority of diabetic patients.

Fewer than 5% of diabetics are Type 1. The total destruction of insulin-producing cells in the pancreas is the underlying cause for Type 1 diabetes. However, as they age, many Type 1 diabetics also suffer from insulin resistance. Therefore, all Type 1 diabetics should pay close attention to this discussion of insulin resistance. Toward the end of this chapter, I will also discuss what causes Type 1 diabetes in more detail.

Insulin Resistance Syndrome

Insulin Resistance Syndrome is the most common medical condition affecting the world today. It is estimated that well over 100 million Americans have it and don't know it. Worldwide, there is an epidemic of this devastating disease. And most people have never heard of it.

For a long time we have known that obesity, high blood pressure, and cholesterol disorder tend to cluster in a person who subsequently develops Type 2 diabetes or has a heart attack or stroke. What we didn't know was the link between these medical conditions. In the last twenty years, there has been tremendous research in this field. Now we know the missing link is insulin resistance, hence the name Insulin Resistance Syndrome.

Insulin Resistance Syndrome (IRS) is also known as metabolic syndrome or syndrome X. I prefer Insulin Resistance Syndrome because it clearly defines the underlying disease process. Syndrome X sounds to me like the title of a Hollywood movie: catchy, but ultimately a bit confusing. Metabolic syndrome does not fully convey the serious nature of this condition, either.

The Major Components of Insulin Resistance Syndrome (IRS)

The major components of Insulin Resistance Syndrome include:

- Being overweight, especially around the waistline; this is also called abdominal obesity (a waistline of more than 35 inches in females and more than 40 inches in males; in Asians, these numbers are 32 and 35 inches respectively)
- Low HDL cholesterol (less than 50 mg/dl in females; less than 40 mg/dl in males)
- High triglycerides (more than 150 mg/dl)
- High blood pressure (more than 130/85 mm Hg, even in a physician's office)

- Impaired glucose tolerance (blood glucose between 140 mg/dl and 200 mg/dl at two hours after 75 grams of a glucose drink in an oral glucose tolerance test*)
- Impaired fasting glucose (a fasting blood glucose level between 100 mg/dl and 125 mg/dl). Many people with impaired fasting glucose or impaired glucose tolerance eventually develop diabetes. Therefore, these conditions are also known as prediabetes.
- Diabetes (a fasting blood glucose level of more than 125 mg/dl or a two-hour blood glucose level of more than 200 mg/dl in an oral glucose tolerance test)
- Increased tendency for clot formation, which can cause an acute heart attack or stroke
- High insulin level in the blood
- Increased uric acid level in the blood (which can cause gout)
- Fatty liver (an abnormal deposition of fat in the liver that can cause liver dysfunction)
- Women with Polycystic Ovary Syndrome (PCO syndrome); symptoms include irregular menses, excessive facial hair growth, and acne

You don't have to have all of these conditions to fit the diagnosis of Insulin Resistance Syndrome. Most individuals with IRS have abdominal obesity, low HDL cholesterol, and high triglycerides. In more advanced stages of insulin resistance, patients also develop high blood pressure and prediabetes or diabetes.

What combination of these metabolic disorders you have depends upon the severity and duration of insulin resistance in your body and your body's ability to produce large amounts of insulin to meet the challenge of insulin resistance. Some people have a

---

* See chapter 3 for details on oral glucose tolerance test.

limited ability to produce large amounts of insulin. These patients usually develop diabetes at a younger age—in their thirties
and forties or even in their teens. Others have an extraordinary
ability to produce large amounts of insulin. These patients do not
develop diabetes until late in life. They may die of a heart attack
or stroke before they develop diabetes.

These metabolic disorders also cluster in family members. For
example, a mother may have high blood pressure while her son
may have diabetes and suffered a heart attack. An aunt may have
diabetes and her niece may have high blood pressure and low
HDL cholesterol.

Initially, people with IRS don't have any symptoms and therefore are under the impression that there is nothing wrong with
them. Then one day, they show up in the emergency room of a
hospital with an acute heart attack. Family and friends wonder
how it could have happened to such a (seemingly) healthy person.

The Causes of Insulin Resistance Syndrome

The main reasons people develop Insulin Resistance Syndrome are:

- Genetic predisposition
- Obesity
- Aging
- Lack of exercise
- Stress

Genetics play an important role in determining the degree of insulin resistance. While no one is immune to this syndrome, certain ethnic groups, such as Native American Indians, African
Americans, Latinos, and Asians, have a higher prevalence of insulin resistance than Caucasians. Make no mistake though. Large

numbers of Caucasians also suffer from this disease. Asians often develop this syndrome even at a relatively normal weight. One in four Latinos is diagnosed with diabetes by the age of forty-five.

Abdominal obesity is a key player in most patients with Insulin Resistance Syndrome, especially in younger individuals. Obesity and diabetes have increased at an alarming rate in the last decade. According to recent statistics from the Centers for Disease Control (CDC), the prevalence of obesity in the U.S. increased by 61% from 1991 to 2000. During the same period, diabetes increased by 49% with a 76% increase in people aged thirty to thirty-nine, according to a study published in 2001 in the *Journal of the American Medical Association.*[1] Obesity in children and adolescents is also rapidly increasing. Children as young as five have exhibited signs of insulin resistance.

As we age, insulin resistance worsens. That is why diabetes, high blood pressure, heart disease, and stroke are so prevalent in people over the age of fifty. In the U.S., seniors are the most rapidly expanding segment of society, which is contributing to the fast rate at which insulin resistance is increasing. Forty percent of adult Americans suffer from Insulin Resistance Syndrome, according to estimates published in 2003 in the *Endocrine Practice,* the official journal of the American College of Endocrinology and the American Association of Clinical Endocrinologists.[2] This number increases to 50% by age seventy. In other words, every other American over the age of seventy has Insulin Resistance Syndrome. These estimates are rather conservative due to the methodology used. In real life, this disease is even more prevalent.

Lack of exercise is another major factor that causes worsening of insulin resistance. Too many of us have become couch potatoes, glued to the ever-present television or computer. The only workout we get is from pressing the remote control for the television or maneuvering the mouse on our computer. Our lifestyles have become too sedentary. An interesting study was published in the *Archives of Internal Medicine* in 2001.[3] The investigators studied 37,918 men between the ages of forty and seventy-five over a period of ten years and found that the risk for development of diabetes was directly related to time spent watching television.

Stress plays a major role in the worsening of insulin resistance. Stress directly causes an increase in two hormones in the body, cortisol and catecholamines. Both of these hormones worsen insulin resistance. People who are stressed (as most of us are to some extent) often overeat despite knowing the health hazards of obesity. Increase in weight further worsens insulin resistance. This is how stress indirectly affects insulin resistance.

Think of insulin resistance as five guys controlling a speeding train. All five of them must halt to stop the deadly train called Insulin Resistance Syndrome. Unfortunately, two out of the five (genetics and aging) are out of your control. That is the reason why diet, exercise, and stress management alone are generally inadequate to prevent diabetes and the other complications of Insulin Resistance Syndrome. You need to add vitamins and drugs to effectively treat this deadly disease.

Insulin Resistance and How It Damages Your Body

There is a tremendous amount of clinical evidence to show that insulin resistance is the root cause for coronary artery disease, stroke, diabetes, and high blood pressure. Insulin resistance causes narrowing of the blood vessels throughout your body. In the heart, it leads to heart attacks; in the brain, it causes stroke and dementia; and in the legs, it causes poor circulation and, ultimately, amputation.

Insulin has several actions in the body, one of which is to drive glucose from the blood into the muscle cells, where it is used as a fuel for energy. Recall the image from chapter 1 of the cell as a small room and a blood vessel as a hallway outside of the room. Glucose, the delivery person, moves through the hallway but is unable to enter the room because the door is closed. Insulin works as the doorman, opening the door for glucose to enter the cell. In individuals with insulin resistance, the door hinges of the cell are rusty, making it difficult for insulin to open the door easily. Now, instead of one doorman, you need three or four. This is insulin resistance. Your body produces excessive insulin to compensate for the door's resistance.

A high level of insulin may keep your blood glucose normal, but is not good for the rest of your body. A high level of insulin causes high blood pressure. This association between high insulin levels and the development of high blood pressure has been confirmed by several researchers.[4]

A high level of insulin is also associated with a high risk for heart disease. This association has been documented by several excellent clinical studies—The Helenski Policeman Study[5], the Paris Prospective Study[6], and the Danish Study.[7]

How does insulin cause heart disease? Insulin stimulates smooth muscle cell growth in the walls of arteries and causes thickening and stiffness of arterial walls, which, in turn, contributes to narrowing of blood vessels.[8] Hypertension (high blood pressure) itself causes further narrowing of the blood vessels. Narrowed blood vessels lead to heart attacks and strokes.

A high level of insulin also leads to the growth of tumors in the body. Several clinical studies have shown a high prevalence of cancer in people with Insulin Resistance Syndrome. Certain cancers, especially breast cancer, colon cancer, and prostate cancer have been linked to insulin resistance. An excellent, large clinical study, known as the American Nurses Health Study was published in *Diabetes Care* in 2003.[9] In this study, 111,488 American female nurses who were thirty to fifty-five years old and free of cancer in 1976 were followed through 1996 for the occurrence of Type 2 diabetes and through 1998 for breast cancer. Women with Type 2 diabetes (a component of Insulin Resistance Syndrome) were found to have a higher incidence of breast cancer than those who did not have diabetes.

As long as your pancreas can churn out lots of extra insulin, your blood glucose will remain in the normal range. This "overworked pancreas" scenario can go on for years in apparently healthy individuals. This phenomenon was brilliantly studied in nondiabetic children of diabetic parents and published in 1990 in the *Annals of Internal Medicine.*[10]

Eventually, your pancreas can't continue to produce large amounts of insulin to compensate for rising insulin resistance. What causes this decline in insulin production by the pancreas is undergoing intense research at this time. We know that genetics play a significant role. Free fatty acids (a product from the breakdown of fat) have also been shown to cause damage to the insulin producing cells (beta cells) of the pancreas.[11]

Once insulin production by the pancreas starts to decline, your blood glucose levels start rising, initially only after meals. This stage is known as impaired glucose tolerance (IGT). At this stage, your fasting blood glucose is usually normal. Impaired glucose tolerance can only be diagnosed if you have an oral glucose tolerance test.

Several years later, your blood glucose starts rising even in the fasting state. This occurs due to insulin resistance in the liver.

Normally your liver produces glucose during a fasting state, such as at night time. Insulin keeps this glucose production in check. However, when there is resistance to the action of insulin, this glucose production by the liver gets into high gear and your fasting blood glucose starts to rise.

If your fasting blood glucose rises into the range of 100–125 mg/dl, it is known as impaired fasting glucose (IFG).

Impaired glucose tolerance and impaired fasting glucose are early stages in the development of diabetes and, therefore, are also known as prediabetes.

Ultimately, a diagnosis of diabetes is made when your fasting blood glucose is more than 125 mg/dl or when your blood glucose is more than 200 mg/dl two hours after a glucose drink in an oral glucose tolerance test.

Another role that insulin plays is to keep fat where it belongs: inside fat cells. In individuals with abdominal obesity, there is resistance to the action of insulin at the level of the fat cells. Consequently, an increased amount of fat escapes from the fat cells and enters the blood stream. A breakdown product of this fat is free fatty acids. Thus, in individuals with insulin resistance, there is a high level of free fatty acids in the blood. The liver takes up these free fatty acids and converts them into VLDL cholesterol (very low density lipoproteins). These cholesterol particles are rich in triglycerides, which is why individuals with insulin resistance have a high level of triglycerides.

When VLDL particles interact with HDL (good cholesterol) particles, VLDL exchanges its triglycerides for the cholesterol of HDL particles. This results in a decrease in HDL cholesterol. These triglycerides-enriched HDL particles also break down easily, which further lowers HDL levels. That is why individuals with insulin resistance end up with low HDL cholesterol.

HDL cholesterol is popularly known as the good cholesterol as it sweeps out the built-up gunk (technically known as plaque) inside the blood vessels. If your HDL is low, you have a decreased number of "sweepers," which means less cleansing and, therefore, more gunk buildup inside your blood vessels. This leads to narrowing of the blood vessels.

VLDL particles also give rise to the formation of another cholesterol particle, known as IDL (intermediate density lipoprotein), which then converts to LDL (low density lipoproteins). LDL particles in individuals with insulin resistance are of Type B, which means that they are small, dense, and get deposited in the walls of blood vessels more easily and are, therefore, more harmful. LDL, VLDL, and IDL particles deposit in the arterial wall and cause narrowing of the vessel wall.

On average, many years of insulin resistance go by before a diagnosis of diabetes is made. During this time, narrowing of the blood vessels takes place due to low HDL cholesterol, Type B LDL cholesterol, elevated IDL and VLDL cholesterol, high insulin levels, and high blood pressure. Narrowing of the blood vessels leads to heart attacks and strokes. Many people die of a heart attack before they are diagnosed with diabetes. Most people have developed advanced narrowing of the blood vessels by the time they are diagnosed with diabetes.

The Stages of Insulin Resistance Syndrome

Insulin resistance is a continuous disease process that worsens over time. In order for you to understand this disease process, I have divided this syndrome into four stages. This staging system is very practical and physicians can easily use it in their day-to-day practice.

Zaidi Staging System of Insulin Resistance Syndrome (IRS)

Stage 1 of IRS	Stage 2 of IRS	Stage 3 of IRS	Stage 4 of IRS
• HDL cholesterol is low • Triglyceride level is high • Insulin level is high • Blood glucose is normal in the fasting state as well as after the glucose intake in the oral glucose tolerance test • Blood pressure is normal	• HDL cholesterol is low • Triglyceride level is high • Insulin level is high • Fasting blood glucose is normal, but blood glucose is elevated in the range of 140–200 mg/dl at two hours in an oral glucose tolerance test; this is known as impaired glucose tolerance (IGT) • Blood pressure is usually high	• HDL cholesterol is low • Triglyceride level is high • Insulin level is high • Fasting blood glucose is elevated in the range of 100–125 mg/dl, which is known as impaired fasting glucose (IFG) • Blood pressure is usually high	• HDL cholesterol is low • Triglyceride level is high • Insulin level is normal to high • Fasting blood glucose is more than 125 mg/dl, which is diagnostic for diabetes • Blood pressure is usually high
At risk for heart attack, stroke, dementia, cancer, fatty liver, and leg amputation High risk for diabetes	High risk for heart attack, stroke, dementia, cancer, fatty liver, and leg amputation; moderate risk for peripheral neuropathy Even higher risk for diabetes	Even higher risk for heart attack, stroke, dementia, cancer, fatty liver, and leg amputation; high risk for peripheral neuropathy Much higher risk for diabetes Many individuals are found to be diabetic on an oral glucose tolerance test	Extremely high risk for heart attack, stroke, dementia, cancer, fatty liver, leg amputation, diabetic neuropathy, eye disease, and kidney disease About 50% of patients have developed diabetic complications at this stage of the disease

Please note that people in stage 1 have normal blood pressure. It is in stage 2, 3, and 4 that blood pressure is high. Therefore, by the time you're found to have high blood pressure, the process of insulin resistance and, consequently, narrowing of the blood vessels, has already been going on for a few years.

Also note that diabetes can be diagnosed at an earlier stage (stage 3) by an oral glucose tolerance test (see chapter 3), as compared to the routine fasting blood glucose test, which diagnoses diabetes at a later, more advanced stage (stage 4). Unfortunately, it is in stage 4 that diabetes is usually diagnosed, because many physicians do not order an oral glucose tolerance test. Therefore, by the time a person is diagnosed with diabetes, the process of insulin resistance and, consequently, narrowing of the blood vessels, has been going on for a very long period of time, usually ten to fifteen years. That is the reason why diabetics are at such a high risk for heart attack, stroke, dementia, kidney failure, blindness, cancer, fatty liver, and amputation of the legs.

Stage 1 of Insulin Resistance Syndrome

In this stage of Insulin Resistance Syndrome, you are a healthy person on the surface. You will pass an annual physical checkup. Your blood pressure, blood glucose, total cholesterol, and LDL (bad) cholesterol are in the normal range. The only abnormality is low HDL (good) cholesterol and high triglycerides. Many laboratories have set their normal ranges too low for HDL cholesterol and too high for triglycerides. Therefore, mild abnormalities of HDL cholesterol and triglycerides are often erroneously placed in the normal column on your blood report. A typical blood cholesterol profile may look like this:

Total cholesterol = 195 mg/dl

LDL cholesterol = 117 mg/dl

Stage 1 IRS

At the age of forty-four, Jeff, an Asian male, started taking Lipitor to control his cholesterol disorder. Over several years, his triglycerides had been in the 200–250 mg/dl range, his HDL cholesterol had been in the 35–45 mg/dl range, and his LDL cholesterol had been in the 130–160 mg/dl range.

Otherwise, he was in excellent health. He was about 10 lbs overweight around his waistline. His blood pressure was normal.

His mother had hypertension. She suffered a debilitating stroke at the age of fifty-five and spent the last twenty-four years of her life wheelchair bound. His father had hypertension and diabetes. One of his brothers developed diabetes at the age of forty-five.

Jeff underwent a two-hour oral glucose tolerance test along with a measurement of his C-peptide level. His blood glucose was normal, but his C-peptide was markedly elevated.

With proper treatment, his C-peptide came down. Seven years later, his blood glucose and blood pressure continue to be normal. With early diagnosis and proper treatment, we halted the progression of his insulin resistance.

Triglycerides = 190 mg/dl

HDL cholesterol = 39 mg/dl

Typically, you will be told that you are in good shape, but in truth, you have Insulin Resistance Syndrome. Narrowing of the blood vessels is developing insidiously. Then one day, out of the blue, you have a heart attack! I have seen these cases too often, and it's one of the reasons I decided to write this book. *Do not ignore* your low HDL cholesterol and high triglycerides. These are early markers for IRS.

If you have the kind of cholesterol profile mentioned above, you should undergo a two-hour oral glucose tolerance test with a measurement of insulin level (or C-peptide). If you are in the early stages of Insulin Resistance Syndrome, your blood glucose levels may be in the normal range, but your insulin levels (or C-peptide) will likely be high, indicating that glucose levels are being kept normal because you are able to produce large amounts of insulin. This large amount of insulin, along with low HDL cholesterol, cause narrowing of the blood vessels.

Even at this early stage, you are at high risk for developing diabetes.

Stage 2 Insulin Resistance Syndrome

Your cholesterol profile is the same as in stage 1, but now you have high blood pressure. Unfortunately, this is often ignored and blamed on being in the doctor's office. ("If you hadn't made me wait forty-five minutes and weren't wearing that scary look-ing white coat, my blood pressure would be just fine, doc!") If the stress of being in a doctor's office causes your blood pressure to rise, just think what happens in your everyday life when you get stuck in a traffic jam or misplace your wallet. Life is full of stresses everyday. Any blood pressure higher than 130/85 mm Hg/, even in a doctor's office, is too high. A good blood pressure is less than 115/75 mm Hg.

In this stage, you also have impaired glucose tolerance (IGT) that is diagnosed only if you have an oral glucose tolerance test. IGT is also known as prediabetes. Your risk for progression to diabetes is very high.

Remember, your fasting blood glucose is normal at this stage. You are generally given a clean bill of health. But in fact, the process of narrowing your blood vessels is getting worse. Your impending date in the hospital emergency room is looming.

At this stage, many people develop tingling and numbness of toes (and sometimes fingers) as a manifestation of peripheral

Stage 2 IRS

At the age of seventy-one, Zack, a Caucasian male, developed tingling in his fingertips. For many years, his HDL cholesterol was low and his blood pressure was high.

During a two-hour oral glucose tolerance test (OGTT), Zack's fasting blood glucose was normal at 90 mg/dl, but at one hour, it climbed to 232 mg/dl, and at two hours, it was still high at 154 mg/dl. This indicated that he had impaired glucose tolerance (IGT). He was in stage 2 of IRS.

Even at stage 2, Zack had developed peripheral neuropathy manifesting as tingling in his fingertips. In addition, he had also developed severe narrowing of his coronary arteries, which had required heart bypass surgery three years before.

neuropathy. Unfortunately, you are told you don't have diabetes because your fasting blood glucose is normal. You undergo an extensive diagnostic workup to find out the reason for your peripheral neuropathy and often no reason is found. You and your physician get totally confused and frustrated. One simple test, the oral glucose tolerance test, would easily diagnose your condition. Unfortunately, this important test is rarely done.

Stage 3 Insulin Resistance Syndrome

In stage 3, you will have the same cholesterol profile as in stage 1, and you will have high blood pressure. In addition, now your fasting blood glucose has escalated into the range of 100–125 mg/dl. You now have impaired fasting glucose (IFG).

Many patients in this stage could be diagnosed with diabetes if they have an oral glucose tolerance test.

Narrowing of the blood vessels has advanced even further. You are at an even higher risk for heart attack, stroke, dementia, and peripheral neuropathy.

Stage 3 IRS

Miley, a seventy-eight-year-old Asian female, consulted me for her elevated serum triglycerides level. Her medical records showed that two years prior, her serum triglyceride level was elevated at 520 mg/dl and her fasting blood glucose was elevated at 112 mg/dl. Her physician placed her on Lipitor, but she continued to have elevated triglycerides. She was amazed when I told her that her blood glucose was in the range of prediabetes. She complained of tingling and numbness in her toes that had been gradually worsening over the past several years.

Her mother had Type 2 diabetes.

Mylie was overweight around her waistline. Her blood pressure was high at 130/90 mm Hg.

I ordered a two-hour oral glucose tolerance test (OGTT) with the following results.

	Baseline	One hour	Two hours
Blood Glucose	112 mg/dl	243 mg/dl	234 mg/dl

Her fasting blood glucose was elevated into the range of IFG, putting her into stage 3 of IRS. With the help of the OGTT, we were able to diagnose her diabetes. At this stage, IRS had already caused peripheral neuropathy in the form of tingling and numbness of her toes.

Stage 4 Insulin Resistance Syndrome

With stage 4 IRS, you have the same cholesterol profile as in stage 1 and you have high blood pressure. In addition, now your fasting blood glucose is above 125 mg/dl. You are now officially diabetic. Unfortunately, you may be told that "you have borderline high blood sugar" or "you have a touch of diabetes." You might even be told to "cut sugar out of your diet and everything will be all right." The fact is that the narrowing of your blood

Stage 4 IRS

Danny, a forty-five-year-old Caucasian male, came to see me because his sister read about Insulin Resistance Syndrome and insisted that he be evaluated for it. He thought he was in good health. For a long time, he had low HDL cholesterol and high triglycerides. He also had high blood pressure, but it was written off as caused by the stress of being in a doctor's office.

On my evaluation, he was obese, especially around his stomach. His blood pressure was high at 150/100 mm Hg. His HDL cholesterol was low at 34 mg/dl and his triglycerides level was high at 646 mg/dl. I ordered an oral glucose tolerance test, which showed that he had developed diabetes. His insulin level was also high.

Results of the two-hour oral glucose tolerance test:

	Baseline	One hour	Two Hours
Blood Glucose	129 mg/dl	283 mg/dl	238 mg/dl

OGTT results clearly showed that he was a diabetic. He was a ticking time bomb. Amazingly, he believed nothing was wrong with him. I diagnosed him with Insulin Resistance Syndrome, stage 4, and started the appropriate treatment. He is enjoying "true" good health now.

vessels is very advanced and your risk for heart attack, stroke, dementia, and peripheral neuropathy is extremely high.

The Risk Profile for Insulin Resistance Syndrome

Chances are that you have Insulin Resistance Syndrome if you are/have any three of the following:

- Older than forty years old

- Family history of diabetes, high blood pressure, cholesterol disorder, heart attack, stroke, or dementia
- Overweight, especially in the abdominal area, with a waistline of more than 35 inches if you are a woman or more than 40 inches if you are man (for Asians, these numbers are 32 inches and 35 inches respectively)
- A sedentary lifestyle
- HDL cholesterol of less than 50 mg/dl for females; less than 40 mg/dl for males
- Triglyceride level greater than 150 mg/dl
- High blood pressure (higher than 130/85 mm Hg, even in a physician's office)
- Fasting blood glucose of more than 100 mg/dl but less than 125 mg/dl (this is known as impaired fasting glucose)
- Impaired glucose tolerance (IGT) diagnosed on a two-hour oral glucose tolerance test
- Diabetes
- Heart attack, angioplasty, or heart bypass surgery
- Stroke or ministroke
- Dementia
- History of gestational diabetes or delivery of a baby that weighs more than 9 lbs
- Women with polycystic ovary syndrome (most common cause for irregular menses, acne, and excessive facial hair)
- Abnormal liver function due to fatty liver in the absence of alcoholism and hepatitis

Laboratory Testing for Insulin Resistance Syndrome

The following three blood tests can appropriately diagnose Insulin Resistance Syndrome in most people:

Blood Test for Low HDL Cholesterol and High Triglyceride Level

Low HDL Cholesterol	Less than 50 mg/dl in women Less than 40 mg/dl in men	Regardless of lab reference Range
High Triglyceride level	Greater than 150 mg/dl	Regardless of lab reference Range

Low HDL cholesterol and/or high triglycerides strongly indicate that you are at risk of having Insulin Resistance Syndrome, in spite of what the lab may say is a safe range.

Oral Glucose Tolerance Test (OGTT)

This test can appropriately diagnose impaired glucose tolerance (IGT), impaired fasting glucose (IFG), as well as diabetes, which are various stages in the progression of Insulin Resistance Syndrome. See chapter 3 for details on the oral glucose tolerance test.

Blood Insulin Level or C-peptide Level

An elevated blood insulin level (or C-peptide level) strongly indicates that you have Insulin Resistance Syndrome.

Why the Diagnosis of IRS Is Important

Insulin Resistance Syndrome in its early stages usually does not cause any symptoms. However, it gradually causes narrowing of the blood vessels, which is known as atherosclerosis. Patients with atherosclerosis are at high risk for heart attacks, strokes, dementia, and leg amputation. These patients are also at a very high risk for development of prediabetes and diabetes, which predisposes them to additional complications, including kidney disease, blindness, and peripheral neuropathy of the feet and hands. In addition, these patients are at a high risk for cancer and liver dysfunction. Early diagnosis and proper treatment of Insulin Resistance Syndrome can prevent these hideous complications.

If diagnosed at the stage of prediabetes, these patients can prevent the development of diabetes.

Patients who undergo coronary angioplasty or heart bypass surgery usually have Insulin Resistance Syndrome as the underlying cause. If insulin resistance is not diagnosed and treated appropriately (which unfortunately happens a lot), these patients end up requiring repeated angioplasties. Many end up having bypass surgery.

It is only when Insulin Resistance Syndrome is properly diagnosed and treated that patients are safe from further complications. Then they don't need repeated angioplasties. They don't suffer from stroke, dementia, and diabetes. They can prevent kidney failure, blindness, and leg amputation.

Why Insulin Resistance Syndrome Isn't Diagnosed

Over the years, I have seen several thousand patients with Insulin Resistance Syndrome. To my surprise, few have heard of Insulin Resistance Syndrome. It's not that they haven't seen physicians before. Often they have seen several physicians, including cardiologists, as many have undergone coronary angioplasties. Upon reviewing their old medical records, I find that they have had low HDL cholesterol, high triglycerides, high blood pressure, and elevated fasting blood glucose values for years. Insulin Resistance Syndrome was obvious, but no physician had diagnosed it. To me, it's a very frustrating and sad situation.

Lester, a forty-two-year-old Caucasian male, came to see me out of desperation. At the age of thirty-six, he had heart bypass surgery. Six years later, he started having chest pain again. His cardiologist discovered that even his bypass grafts had shut down. There was near complete blockage of all three major coronary arteries. Angioplasty was attempted but unsuccessful. He was told that the prognosis was grim. He had about six months to live. At that point, his wife (who happened to be my patient) brought him to see me.

A review of his recent laboratory tests showed that Lester's fasting blood glucose was elevated at 122 mg/dl, which was consistent with the diagnosis of impaired fasting glucose.

His HDL cholesterol was low at 33 mg/dl and his triglyceride level was elevated at 224 mg/dl. His LDL cholesterol was appropriately low at 61 mg/dl due to his drug therapy with Lipitor. His total cholesterol was 139 mg/dl.

Lester's brother died of a heart attack at the age of forty-two. His mother, who had Type 2 diabetes, died of a heart attack at the age of seventy. His father died of a stroke at the age of seventy.

I diagnosed Lester with IRS stage 3 and started him on the appropriate treatment seven years ago. Not only is he still alive, but he's enjoying a good quality of life.

I have given serious consideration to the question of why many physicians fail to diagnose Insulin Resistance Syndrome. Let me share my thoughts and observations with you. The discovery of Insulin Resistance Syndrome is relatively new. Many physicians don't fully understand this syndrome, although these days you can't pick up a medical journal without reading about it. Physicians are stuck in the past and simply continue to practice the way they always have. Like most of us, they are creatures of habit. Unfortunately, in this case, they are creatures of bad habits. They continue to think of obesity, high blood pressure, cholesterol disorder, glucose abnormalities, heart disease, and stroke as separate entities. They don't understand that these medical conditions are linked together with the common thread of one disease process: insulin resistance.

When most physicians look at their obese patients, they don't think of Insulin Resistance Syndrome. To them, obesity is just a weight issue and that is it. They advise their patients to go on a diet and that is the end of the story.

The focus on obesity often stresses cosmetic issues, rather than focusing on health issues. Plastic surgeons will be happy to do liposuction so you can look better but won't tell you anything about insulin resistance. Most insurance companies don't even recognize obesity as a disease state and therefore don't pay for weight management strategies.

The media has done a horrible job in educating the public about Insulin Resistance Syndrome. Everybody keeps hammering on the rise of obesity in this country without ever mentioning Insulin Resistance Syndrome.

When it comes to cholesterol, the general emphasis is on total cholesterol and LDL cholesterol. Physicians often ignore abnormal values of HDL cholesterol and triglycerides. They don't realize that a low HDL cholesterol and/or high triglycerides level indicates Insulin Resistance Syndrome and needs more thorough evaluation.

High blood pressure, in the early stages, often goes untreated because patients generally feel fine and don't want to accept that something is wrong with their health—they are in denial. "Why fix it if it ain't broke" is their mind-set, and many physicians go along with this strategy. Physicians don't realize that high blood pressure indicates the more sinister underlying disease process of insulin resistance. Deadly complications can be prevented if these conditions are treated aggressively in the beginning. The strategy should be to "nip the evil in the bud."

Glucose abnormalities often go unnoticed, and appropriate testing for these abnormalities is often not done. Impaired glucose tolerance is diagnosed on an oral glucose tolerance test, but most physicians don't order this test, relying, instead, on the routine testing of fasting blood glucose. That is why this important diagnosis is often missed. Even an elevation in fasting blood glucose remains under the radar of many physicians and doesn't get their attention.

In my clinical experience, often a patient has fasting blood glucose in a normal range but is found to have impaired glucose tolerance or even full-blown diabetes when the oral glucose tolerance test is given. In other words, impaired glucose tolerance or even diabetes will be missed if the oral glucose tolerance test is not done.

The Cause of Type 1 Diabetes

Type 1 diabetes occurs as a result of the total destruction of beta cells (the insulin producing cells) in the pancreas. This destruction of beta cells in the pancreas takes place because your own immune system has gone wild.

Normally your immune system recognizes anything foreign in your body, such as a virus, and gets rid of it. In patients who ultimately develop Type 1 diabetes, the immune system mistakenly thinks that the beta cells of your pancreas don't belong to you and, therefore, must be destroyed. So it starts attacking the beta cells of your own pancreas. Basically, your own immune system turns against you. That is why we call it an autoimmune disorder.

Gradually beta cells start dying out and insulin production starts declining. Ultimately, there is very little or no insulin production. At that point, you must have the administration of insulin to survive. If Type 1 diabetic patients don't receive insulin, they can rapidly lapse into a coma. They can die if proper treatment is not initiated in time.

Why does the immune system turn against itself and start attacking the beta cells of the pancreas? The exact answer is not entirely clear but here are some explanations.

Some individuals are genetically predisposed to this immune destruction of the beta cells, but this process has to be triggered by some factor in the environment. The possible triggering factors include a viral illness, childhood immunizations, baby formula, preservatives in food, pesticides, and other unrecognized environmental factors. Stress also plays an important role in weakening the immune system.

Patients with Type 1 diabetes are also at high risk for other autoimmune disorders that include:

- Autoimmune thyroid disease, which can result in an underactive thyroid (also known as Hashimoto's thyroiditis) or an overactive thyroid (also known as Grave's disease)
- Impairment of vitamin B12 absorption from the intestines, resulting in vitamin B12 deficiency that may manifest as pernicious anemia; weakness, tingling, and numbness of toes and fingers; unbalanced gait; and dementia
- Autoimmune adrenalitis resulting in adrenal failure (also known as Addison's disease), manifesting as severe fatigue and low blood pressure
- Autoimmune oophoritis resulting in premature menopause
- Lupus and Rheumatoid arthritis

CHAPTER 3

Diagnosing Diabetes

Since the early stages of diabetes usually don't cause any symptoms, diagnosis is often delayed until complications of diabetes are present, most of which are not reversible. So the earlier you get a diagnosis, the better. However, that also means you need to go *looking* for diabetes and not wait until it blindsides you with a heart attack or stroke.

Are you one of the millions of Americans at risk for developing diabetes?

Current estimates indicate that more than 20 million Americans have diabetes and more than 42 million have prediabetes. Around the world, the statistics are equally grim. In 1985 an estimated 30 million people worldwide had diabetes. By 2000, the numbers had increased to 150 million. It is estimated to rise to 333 million by the year 2025.

This explosive increase in the number of diabetics is due to the fact that the major factors causing diabetes—weight gain, lack of exercise, and aging—are increasing.

According to statistics from the Centers for Disease Control (CDC), the prevalence of obesity in the U.S. increased by 61% from 1991 to 2000. During the same period, diabetes increased by 49% with a 76% increase in people aged thirty to thirty-nine, according to a study published in 2001 in the *Journal of the American Medical Association*.[1] Now 14% of U.S. children and adolescents are overweight.

The problem of lack of exercise has worsened with our technological advances. Television has turned us into couch potatoes. Computers have taken over our workplace as well as our leisure activities. The only sports many teenagers play are virtual sports through video games.

And we now know that people over the age of sixty are the most rapidly expanding segment of our society. Aging baby boomers guarantee that the number of seniors will continue to rise for many years to come.

As my patient Margo once said, "Hey, if fat, lazy, and old means I got diabetes, you better haul in everyone from my Tuesday night bingo and get them tested, too!"

Margo was only partially right, because the truth is you don't need to be fat, lazy, or old to get diabetes. But if you are all three, it's definitely time to get tested!

Those at Risk for Developing Diabetes

People with the following characteristics are at high risk for developing Type 2 diabetes and, therefore, should undergo testing for diabetes even if they have no symptoms. Remember, diabetes is a silent killer.

- Older than forty years old
- Family history of diabetes, high blood pressure, cholesterol disorder, heart attack, or stroke
- Overweight, especially in the abdominal area (waistline more than 35 inches in females and 38 inches in males; for

Asians, these numbers are 32 inches in females and 35 inches in males, respectively)
- High blood pressure (greater than 130/85 mm Hg, even in a physician's office)
- Triglyceride level greater than 150 mg/dl
- HDL cholesterol less than 40 mg/dl in males and less than 50 mg/dl in females
- A personal history of heart attack, angioplasty, stent placement, or heart bypass surgery
- A personal history of stroke, ministrokes, or dementia
- A personal history of gestational diabetes or delivery of a baby that weighs more than 9 lbs
- Women with a history of irregular menses, excessive facial hair growth, or acne

When I see any of these features in my patients, I test them for diabetes even if they don't have any symptoms.

The Best Test for the Diagnosis of Diabetes

There are two tests used to diagnose diabetes: the fasting blood glucose (FBG) test and the oral glucose tolerance test (OGTT).

The Fasting Blood Glucose Test

Usually this is done as part of a routine blood test after you have fasted overnight.

Fasting Blood Glucose	Greater than 125 mg/dl	Diabetes
Fasting Blood Glucose	100 mg/dl to 125 mg/dl	Impaired fasting glucose (IFG)

Impaired fasting glucose (IFG) means that you have prediabetes and need further testing with an oral glucose tolerance test.

The Oral Glucose Tolerance Test (OGTT)

This is the best test to diagnose diabetes. After an overnight fast, a blood test is drawn for glucose. Then you are given a drink containing 75 grams of glucose. Another blood test is drawn at one hour and then again at two hours. You do not eat or drink anything else during this two-hour period.

	More than 200 mg/dl	Diabetes
Blood Glucose at Two Hours	Between 140 mg/dl and 200 mg/dl	Impaired glucose tolerance (IGT)
	Between 100 mg/dl and 140 mg/dl	Mild glucose intolerance

In nondiabetics, the glucose value should come back to near baseline after two hours. For example, if your fasting blood glucose was 95 mg/dl, then two hours after drinking the 75 grams of glucose, it should come back to about 95 mg/dl.

The two-hour oral glucose tolerance test (OGTT) has been the international standard to diagnose diabetes for a long time. Most scientific studies about diabetes utilize it as *the* diagnostic test.

Several excellent scientific studies have demonstrated that the oral glucose tolerance test is a superior test for diagnosing diabetes compared to the fasting blood glucose test. One such study, published in June 2002 in *Diabetes Care,* the medical journal of the American Diabetes Association, showed that about 66% of individuals who were found to have diabetes on the two-hour oral glucose tolerance test would have been missed if only the fasting blood glucose was used to diagnose diabetes. Many other studies have shown similar results.[2]

The importance of the oral glucose tolerance test was emphasized in a review article published in 2002 in *Diabetes Care*.[3] Diabetes can be diagnosed about three to five years sooner with the oral glucose tolerance test as compared to the fasting blood glucose test.

A number of excellent studies have also clearly demonstrated that postmeal glucose (i.e. blood glucose level at one and two hours after the glucose drink in the oral glucose tolerance test) is a strong predictor of cardiovascular disease. One such study, The Chicago Heart Study, reported that cardiovascular mortality significantly increased in men whose blood glucose rose to more than 200 mg/dl at one hour after taking the glucose drink in the OGTT. This study was published in *Diabetes Care* in 1997.[4] In another excellent study, the Honolulu Heart Program, 6,394 nondiabetic men, aged forty-five to seventy years old, were given the glucose tolerance test and followed for twelve years for the development of heart disease. The risk for heart disease was directly related to postmeal glucose value: the higher the postmeal glucose, the higher the risk for heart disease. This famous study was published in *Diabetes* in 1987.[5]

A landmark European study known as the DECODE Study clearly showed that a two-hour blood glucose level is a better predictor of death from cardiovascular disease than the fasting blood glucose.[6]

Unfortunately, many physicians do not order this simple but extremely important test. The only reasons cited against the use of the oral glucose tolerance test are its cost and inconvenience. But to my mind, adding a couple of blood draws and a drink of glucose should not have a significant financial impact, especially when you consider the consequences of delayed diagnosis of diabetes. Is it

Betty, a slender sixty-six-year-old Caucasian female, came to me *looking* to rule out diabetes. Her mother and two brothers were diabetic. She had a history of cholesterol disorder.

On a recent routine lab test by her internist, Betty had a high non-fasting blood glucose level of 161 mg/dl. Surprisingly, she was told that it didn't mean anything since it was nonfasting. However, Betty wasn't so sure, so she decided to consult me.

I ordered an oral glucose tolerance test (OGTT). Betty's results were as follows:

	Baseline	*One hour*	*Two hours*
Blood Glucose	109 mg/dl	215 mg/dl	247 mg/dl

Betty's two-hour blood glucose value was consistent with the diagnosis of diabetes, although her fasting glucose was not in the diabetic range. Her diagnosis of diabetes would have been missed if I had not given her the oral glucose tolerance test.

worth a few extra dollars to avoid eye disease, stroke, or a heart attack? Sitting comfortably in an office for two hours to complete the test is hardly a real inconvenience. Compare it to the real inconvenience and unpleasant reality of a routine colonoscopy, rectal exam, mammogram, or pap smear. A couple of blood draws are hardly an inconvenience compared to any one of these procedures.

Sadly, most physicians continue to rely on the fasting blood glucose test to diagnose diabetes. I routinely utilize the oral glucose tolerance test in my clinical practice. I have diagnosed many patients with diabetes who had a normal fasting blood glucose level, a diagnosis that would have been missed if I had not ordered an oral glucose tolerance test. And I have heard few complaints from patients about this test. Most patients are grateful that a diagnosis of diabetes was made early so that complications could be avoided. If you have any of the risk factors for diabetes mentioned above, talk to your doctor about getting an OGTT test.

But My Routine Blood Test Was Normal!

A routine blood test is usually just a *fasting* chemistry panel. As you can see from Betty's example, her fasting blood glucose was not in the "diabetic" range, even though she was diabetic. The fact is that your blood glucose value in the fasting state remains in the normal range for a long period of time, even though you may have early diabetes. The reason is that the development of diabetes does not occur overnight. It is a long, continuous process that develops over a period of years.

Blood glucose after a meal usually rises to a diabetic range long before your fasting blood glucose becomes elevated to the diabetic range. Therefore, a normal blood glucose level on a routine fasting blood test can be misleading and provide a false sense of security. You still might have diabetes!

o o o

Rhonda, a sixty-five-year-old Caucasian female with a history of high blood pressure, cholesterol disorder, obesity, and underactive thyroid, came in for a thyroid checkup. She had gained about 15 lbs over the past several years and complained of fatigue. Her mother had also suffered from high blood pressure.

Medications

Lipitor 20 mg/day
Lotensin 20 mg/day

Physical Examination

Blood pressure = 170/90 mm Hg
Weight = 164 lbs;
Height = 5'2" (approximately 50 lbs overweight)
Abdominal obesity was present

Laboratory Results

Fasting blood glucose = 97mg/dl (normal range 70 mg/dl–100 mg/dl)
Triglycerides = 346 mg/dl (should be less than 150 mg/dl)
HDL cholesterol = 55 mg/dl (should be more than 50 mg/dl in females)
LDL cholesterol = 130 mg/dl (should be less than 130 mg/dl in a nondiabetic)

Diagnosis

I suspected diabetes in this patient because she had the following risk factors for the development of diabetes:

- Older than forty years old
- High blood pressure
- High triglyceride level
- Abdominal obesity
- Family history of high blood pressure

Therefore, I ordered an oral glucose tolerance test (OGTT) with the following results:

	Fasting	One hour	Two hours
Blood Glucose	83 mg/dl	235 mg/dl	216 mg/dl

Her baseline fasting blood glucose was perfectly normal, but at two hours, her blood glucose values were consistent with the diagnosis of diabetes. I would have missed the diagnosis of diabetes if I had relied on just the fasting blood glucose.

The Role of Family History on Diabetes

A common misconception is that if you have no family history of diabetes, then you are safe and immune to the development of diabetes. Unfortunately, that simply isn't true.

You *can* develop diabetes even if you have no family history of diabetes! Diabetes is only one of several components of the underlying disease Insulin Resistance Syndrome. High triglycerides, low HDL cholesterol, high blood pressure, heart attack, stroke, and dementia are some of the other manifestations of Insulin Resistance Syndrome.

Different family members may have different combinations of these manifestations of Insulin Resistance Syndrome. For example, your mother may have high blood pressure and diabetes and now you have low HDL cholesterol. Your aunt may have had a heart attack and now you have high blood pressure. Your grandfather may have suffered a stroke and now you have diabetes.

Other family members may have died from other causes before any component of Insulin Resistance Syndrome developed.

o   o   o

Leonard, a seventy-six-year-old Caucasian male, was referred to me by his neurologist. Leonard had consulted his neurologist for tingling in his toes. For the past five years, an internist had treated Leonard for obesity, high blood pressure, and cholesterol disorder. Leonard's mother had also suffered from high blood pressure.

Diagnosis

Leonard had the following risk factors for the development of diabetes:

- Older than forty years old
- Obesity
- High blood pressure
- Cholesterol disorder
- Positive family history for high blood pressure

The neurologist was well aware of Insulin Resistance Syndrome and ordered an oral glucose tolerance test (OGTT) to screen for diabetes.

The results of the OGTT were as follows:

	Fasting	One hour	Two hours
Blood Glucose	123 mg/dl	305 mg/dl	257 mg/dl

This test confirmed that Leonard had diabetes. His baseline fasting blood glucose was not in the diabetic range, so the diagnosis of diabetes would have been missed if he had not taken the oral glucose tolerance test. A twenty-four-hour urine test showed that he had already developed diabetic kidney disease and that his kidney function was reduced by 50%.

This case again reaffirms that many physicians often miss the diagnosis of diabetes because they only rely on the fasting blood glucose test. Unfortunately, by the time he was diagnosed, Leonard had already developed two major complications of diabetes: kidney disease and nerve disease in his feet. These complications could have been prevented had he been given an oral glucose tolerance test a few years earlier.

CHAPTER 4

The Conventional Treatment for Diabetes and Its Flaws

Betsy, a fifty-five-year-old Caucasian female, came to see me for her uncontrolled Type 2 diabetes that had been diagnosed ten years earlier. Initially, her physician treated her with various sulfonylurea drugs (Micronase, Diabeta, Glucotrol) for a few years. Later, her physician switched her to insulin therapy as these sulfonylurea drugs had failed to control her diabetes. At the time I saw her, she was on 40 units of NPH insulin plus 20 units of regular insulin, in the morning and in the evening. Despite insulin therapy, her diabetes was uncontrolled. She had also developed three major complications of diabetes: heart disease, kidney disease, and peripheral neuropathy. Obviously, she was quite frustrated and demoralized.

Betsy's story is all too common. Most Type 2 diabetic patients start out on oral sulfonylurea medication and in a few years end up on insulin therapy. They often develop devastating complications of diabetes along the way. It's the typical end result of the conventional approach to the treatment of Type 2 diabetes.

Unfortunately, popular literature about diabetes continues to propagate this conventional approach to treatment, and most physicians continue to utilize it. If this is your story, you know all too well that it is you, the patient, who ultimately suffers from this outdated method of treatment. My treatment protocol, outlined in Part II, offers you hope for reversing your diabetic complications or preventing them in the first place. Before getting into the particulars of my approach, however, let's examine the conventional treatment to understand why it is flawed.

The Conventional Treatment Approach

The conventional treatment approach to Type 2 diabetes focuses on controlling blood glucose by any means. After your diagnosis, as you may have already experienced, your physician will recommend that you start a special diet based on calorie counting.

The problems with the typical antidiabetic diet are:

1. The diet permits too many calories
2. No consideration is given to whether you are a Type 1 or Type 2 diabetic
3. No consideration is given to your age—you get the same diet whether you are forty or seventy years old
4. Too many carbohydrates are permitted

Once the diet approach fails to achieve glucose control, you start taking a sulfonylurea drug, such as Glucotrol (glipizide), Diabeta (glyburide), Micronase (glyburide), Glynase (glyburide), or Amaryl (glimepiride). Initially, this sulfonylurea drug controls your blood glucose, but later it starts to fail. Your physician increases the dosage until even the maximum dose of that drug is unable to adequately control your blood glucose. At that point, your physician adds another drug, usually Glucophage (metformin). Initially you may get a little response, but then your blood glucose starts to escalate again. Finally, you might be placed on insulin therapy, the dosage of which keeps increasing in order to control your blood glucose levels. Eventually, you are on a high dose of insulin but your blood glucose is still not adequately controlled. What is more, insulin shots are not only a nuisance for patients, but they also contribute to episodes of low blood sugar, weight gain, and do not treat the root cause of diabetes: insulin resistance!

In medical literature, we call this gradual but inevitable increase in medications the step-up approach—start with one drug, once that fails, add another one and then another and so forth and so on. This step-up approach is marked with one failure after another.

The Step-Up Approach and Its Associated Risks

This conventional step-up treatment considers diabetes to be simply a matter of high blood glucose, and your physician's efforts will be aimed at controlling blood glucose by any means. The problem with this approach is that most diabetics suffer from heart attacks and strokes, despite good control of their blood glucose. This is because conventional treatment of Type 2 diabetes does not treat insulin resistance, the underlying root cause for Type 2 diabetes. Insulin resistance is also the root cause of heart attacks and strokes in diabetic patients. If insulin resistance, the main culprit, remains unchecked, these patients suffer from heart attacks and strokes, despite receiving treatment for their blood glucose. Untreated insulin resistance can also lead to many other complications including dementia, poor leg circulation, impotence, kidney disease, liver dysfunction, and cancer.

Heart Attack

Another serious problem with sulfonylurea drugs is their potential for actually causing an acute heart attack. This was the conclusion of an excellent study carried out in the 1970s. It involved patients at multiple university teaching hospitals in the U.S. and was *not* funded by drug companies. This study, known as UGDP (University Group Diabetes Program), found that diabetic patients on a sulfonylurea drug were 2 1/2 times more likely to suffer a heart attack than those on a restricted diet alone. Unfortunately, physicians continue to use sulfonylurea drugs as the first line of therapy and often the only drug in the initial treatment of Type 2 diabetic patients.

Weight Gain

Sulfonylurea drugs, as well as insulin, cause significant weight gain. Weight gain causes insulin resistance to worsen, requiring an increase in the dose of sulfonylurea and/or insulin to control blood glucose. A vicious cycle sets in, in which the patient keeps gaining weight, blood glucose keeps climbing, and the dosage of drugs keeps escalating. This frustrates both the patient and physician.

Low Blood Sugar

Sulfonylurea drugs and insulin, employed in the conventional treatment strategy, often result in episodes of low blood sugar, which has serious consequences. The symptoms of low blood glucose include cold sweats, palpitations, weakness, a feeling of passing out, dizziness, and foggy thinking. If not treated in time, the patient can lapse into a coma. These symptoms mimic an acute heart attack or stroke.

I vividly remember one night my father-in-law calling frantically that his wife (my mother-in-law) might be having a heart attack. She was just getting over the flu and hadn't eaten much that day but had still taken all of her medications, including her glyburide (a sulfonylurea drug), which can cause low blood sugar. I advised my father-in-law to call 911 and, in the meantime, give her sugar. Fifteen minutes later, I was relieved to hear that my mother-in-law was feeling much better.

Later on, I had to have a serious chat with her physician about the flaws of this *old* treatment strategy and educate him about my new revolutionary approach. Now that my mother-in-law is on my treatment approach, she hasn't had any episodes of low blood sugar! Did I mention that I am now her favorite son-in-law?

As for Betsy, I also placed her on my new treatment approach. She got off insulin shots, reversed her kidney disease, brought her peripheral neuropathy under control, and hasn't had any more heart problems in the last ten years.

PART TWO

TAKING CHARGE OF YOUR DIABETES

CHAPTER 5

The Five Pillars of Treatment

Up until now, I've been talking about what causes diabetes, how diabetes is diagnosed, and what the standard treatments have been. As I've noted, the standard treatment approach to treating Type 2 diabetes—an outdated diet and then a stepping-up of medications—is both out-of-date and dangerous. Let's look now at my new treatment approach, one that I've developed through my clinical practice over the last ten years, and one that I know works! (For treatment recommendations for Type 1 diabetes, see chapter 10.)

My new treatment strategy treats the underlying disease process that causes Type 2 diabetes—insulin resistance—instead of just controlling blood glucose.

Insulin resistance is caused by *five* factors:

1. Obesity
2. Sedentary life style (lack of exercise)
3. Stress
4. Genetics
5. Aging

My new treatment strategy consists of five components. I call these the five pillars of treatment:

1. Diet
2. Exercise
3. Stress management
4. Vitamins
5. Prescription drugs

In the next four chapters, I describe these five pillars in detail. Since exercise is one way to reduce stress, I have combined exercise and stress management in one chapter. You need to focus on all five pillars in order to achieve good control of your diabetes.

CHAPTER 6

Dr. Z's Diabetic Diet

Nothing is more confusing and frustrating for diabetic patients than their diet. There are several reasons for this confusion, and perhaps you'll see your own struggle in this list.

1. *Most physicians do not receive appropriate training in nutrition.* From their residency training days, they remember just one diet recommended for every diabetic patient: an 1800-calories-per-day diabetic diet. Chances are that you will be placed on this famous 1800-calorie diet, whether you are thirty-five or seventy years old, male or female. The truth is that 1800 calories per day is excessive for most people older than forty years old. No wonder many diabetic patients continue to have high blood glucose values.

2. *Many dietitians advocate a diet consisting of three regular meals and three snacks, regardless of diabetes type or treatment.* This diet is usually suitable for Type 1 diabetic patients who are generally young, thin, and on insulin injections. Unfortunately, the same diet is prescribed for Type 2 diabetics who are generally older, obese, and not on insulin.

3. Most dietitians teach you to consume a set number of calories from carbohydrates, fats, and proteins. This is not very practical. Try going to a restaurant and figuring out the percentages of carbohydrates, fat, and protein before you order your food. Good luck! Even when you prepare your food at home, computing the percentages every day is more than most people want to tangle with. Most foods consist of carbohydrates, fats, and proteins in a complex manner. That is why various foods with apparently similar carbohydrate-calorie counts have a significantly different impact on your blood glucose level.

One conclusion is clear: your diet must be individualized. Here's what we do know:

- The appropriate diet for a Type 1 diabetic patient is different from a Type 2 diabetic patient
- The appropriate diet for an obese person is different from that of a lean person
- The appropriate diet for a seventy-year-old patient is different from that of a thirty-year-old patient; daily caloric requirements reduce drastically as we age, especially after the age of fifty
- The appropriate diet for a sedentary person is different from that of an active person
- The appropriate diet for a diabetic patient taking pills is different from the diet of a diabetic on insulin injections; diet will also vary depending upon the type of drugs you take
- The appropriate diet of a Type 2 diabetic on insulin injections is different from a Type 1 diabetic on insulin injections; dietary requirements vary depending on the insulin regimen
- The appropriate diet for a diabetic on an insulin pump is different from a diabetic on insulin injections

Why Most Diets Fail

I'm sure you've resolved many a time to change your diet in order to avoid the horrible diabetic complications your doctor keeps talking about. For a few days or even weeks, you follow your diet diligently. However, eventually you slip up or slack off or give up. Slowly, you gain back all the weight you lost. You're back to square one. Do you ever wonder what really happened? You want to do what's good for your health, but you end up doing what's bad for your health. Crazy, isn't it?

Take heart: diabetics aren't by any means the only category of people who struggle with this issue. Almost everyone sometimes feels as if there's someone else controlling their mind. Most people hear that inner voice that says, "Oh, that wonderful cake. A little piece won't harm me. Life is short, enjoy it." If you obey this inner voice, before you know it, you've finished that piece of cake.

Unfortunately, if you've had trouble sticking to your diet and/or are presently overweight—whether you are diabetic or not—it's likely that this inner voice is largely in control of your eating behavior! It enslaves you. So before you can make any true, everlasting change in your eating pattern, you need to be free from this inner voice. Before you can be free of it, you need to fully understand it.

The inner voice that keeps you off track and off your diet consists of memories, thoughts, and ideas that swirl around in your mind. From your childhood, you learn that pleasure and fun comes from food. Birthday parties, holidays, family get-togethers—at each occasion, food is the center of the celebration. You're encouraged to overeat. Often, this food is unhealthy. Cakes, pies, cookies, donuts, pizza: the list goes on and on. Yet it's all wrapped up in the warm glow of fun and pleasure. As you grow up, you keep adding memories of fun and pleasure through overeating calorie-laden and sugary food. This is how your mind gets conditioned and then controls your eating behavior.

Your inner voice also gets strong feedback from the collective food associations in your particular society or culture. How many times have mothers implored their child to finish the food on their plate because children are starving in other countries? You are told you need to grow up to be big and strong. In many societies, this association holds true, especially for males. The bigger you are, the stronger you are. Sports heroes are often big guys. The more you can eat, the more macho you are.

Restaurants offer buffet deals: eat as much as you want for the same price. Eating contests reward the winner who eats the most. Restaurants brag about the size of their servings—the biggest hamburger in town, etc.

In the workplace, snacking is commonplace. I'm amazed at the amount of food I see at the nurses' station in the hospital. My techie friends tell me they usually have a bag of chips and a can of soda when they're at the computer. Even at physicians' conferences, just after we've had a talk about the epidemic of obesity and diabetes, we take a break for a snack filled with donuts, pastries, and soda.

Often food is an expression of love, respect, and gratitude. Mothers might show their love, for instance, by baking chocolate chip cookies and apple pies. As a grown-up, you'll have a hard time resisting them.

Frequently, you may not be hungry, but you eat to please or be respectful to others. Friends may actually get their feelings hurt if you don't eat their food. Your buddies may badger you to drink a beer with them while watching a football game.

Food is more like an emotional bond between parents and children, between friends and colleagues, and between people of the same culture, geographic location, or religion. If you dare not participate, you're an outcast. Can you even imagine not eating that wonderful Thanksgiving dinner or refusing all those Christmas treats? We all want to blend in, be part of our food-celebrating culture, even if it means damaging our own health.

You were having such a wonderful life, full of parties and food for pleasure, and then one day, diabetes ruined it all. Suddenly, you're told to change everything you've been doing your whole life. Your inner voice says, "No way! We're in this together and I'm not letting you take away all my fun! Listen to me!" This is the main reason you don't adhere to a good eating pattern for more than a few days. You're up against a lifetime of pleasurable, conditioned eating behavior.

So, how do you get freedom from this understandably powerful inner voice? You do it with wisdom. Logic and awareness kills this monster. First of all, become fully aware of where your food associations come from. Take charge of your eating needs instead of letting habit and cultural pressures control your patterns. Use logic. Eat only when you are hungry: not for fun, not for pleasure, not to stuff down your depression. Eat because you are hungry and your body needs food. When you're working on the computer, reading, or watching TV, don't snack. In the grocery store, only buy those foods that are healthy for you. Don't buy food that you know is bad for you. It's during these times of temptation that you need to be fully aware of your triggers. Your inner voice—conditioned as it is from years of eating as you please—will call to you, talk to you, cajole and tempt you. Watch this inner voice with full inner awareness. It's no more than thoughts and emotions. Watch them. But don't get tangled. Don't get involved with them or condemn them. Watch them with a little distance from neutral ground.

Each time you are tempted to indulge—whether at a party, or when you're feeling sad and lonely—be fully aware of the memories and cultural conditioning that is behind your feelings.

There will be setbacks when you lose total control over yourself and finish a half gallon of ice cream in one sitting. The next day, you feel guilty and sad. Low self-esteem crawls in. "I don't have what it takes to stay disciplined. I'm a loser, so I may as well eat some more ice cream."

Don't feel bad and blame yourself. You just got overwhelmed by your inner voice, a voice that is actually not even part of your true self. You acquired it from society, as social conditioning as you grew up. If you stay fully aware of this all the time, that pesky inner voice will start to lose its power over you. Eventually, you'll be in charge of your eating patterns without any effort. Understanding the years of unchecked eating patterns rooted in memories and cultural conditioning is the first—and most important—step toward controlling what you eat.

The Diet for Type 2 Diabetic Patients

In the past, I recommended that patients follow the diabetic dietary guidelines from big medical organizations. Like other physicians, I purchased "Diet for Diabetics" booklets and gave them to my diabetic patients. In addition, I used to refer my diabetic patients to dietitians. But most of my diabetic patients continued to have uncontrolled diabetes.

At every visit, I would remind them to be compliant with diet and medications. They swore they were following all the advice given. Like most physicians, I used to presume they weren't really following the diet.

Then one day, a new thought occurred to me. "Maybe they are following the diet. Maybe the problem is with the diet itself." That was one of those days that changed my perspective about diabetes treatment forever. I started investigating the proper diet for my diabetic patients. After a lot of research and years of testing my theories, I put together a diet that really works for my diabetic patients. In the last ten years, my patients have tremendously benefited from this diet.

On a personal note, I placed myself on this diet although I am not diabetic. I lost about fifteen pounds and reached my ideal body weight. Ten years later, I am still my ideal body weight. Therefore, I recommend this diet to anyone who is overweight.

As I mentioned earlier, there is no one diet that will work for everyone or for every diabetic. My "Dr. Z's Diet" presents guidelines for a typical fifty-year-old Type 2 diabetic who is overweight and not on insulin. Meal suggestions that will help you meet these guidelines—for breakfast, lunch, dinner, and several kinds of take-out or restaurant styles—follow. These guidelines will help you lose weight, and, combined with the exercise, stress management, vitamin supplement, and prescription drug guidelines outlined in the chapters that follow, will help you take charge of your diabetes.

If you're taking insulin, see page 76 for diet recommendations.

Dr. Z's Diet Guidelines

1. No More Than Three Meals a Day

Eat three regular meals per day. Dinner should be the lightest meal of your day and lunch the heaviest. Eat dinner at least three hours before bedtime. Older individuals can try just two meals a day such as breakfast and early dinner. If you feel a little hungry in between meals, try to remember that it is at these times that you are actually burning calories and losing weight. But make sure you don't have low blood sugar (blood sugar of less than 70 mg/dl) at these times by checking your blood glucose level if you feel hungry. See chapter 12 for monitoring guidelines.

2. Reduce the Size of Your Portion

Contrary to your parent's teaching, you don't have to finish all the food on your plate. In fact, learn to leave some food on your plate!

Or use smaller plates. This psychological trick helps with controlling the size of your portion. Serving size is especially huge in American restaurants. In general, when you are eating out, cut the serving in half before you start eating and ask for a doggy bag. This will serve as another meal.

Try to have a garden vegetable salad before lunch and dinner. This serves as a good, low-caloric stomach filler.

Caffeine is a good appetite suppressant. If you have a huge appetite, drink caffeinated tea or coffee about half an hour before your meal to help control your hunger.

3. No Snacks

No snacks, especially when you're watching TV, surfing the Internet, or reading a newspaper. If you have a craving to put something in your mouth, drink black tea or regular coffee. If you absolutely must have a snack, then try something like almonds, cashews, sunflower seeds, popcorn (without butter), pickles, carrot sticks, or other raw vegetables.

4. Cut Carbohydrates

Reduce the amount of bread, rice, and pasta in your diet. Bread includes white bread, whole wheat bread, sourdough bread,

French or Italian bread, donuts, bagels, croissants, pastries, hamburger buns, rolls, pita, pies, Indian naan, tortillas, tacos, enchiladas, and many more similar bakery products. Rice includes white, brown, as well as wild rice.

5. More Proteins and Good Fats

Eat more proteins such as egg whites, lean meat, nonfried chicken, and fish. Other healthy foods include almonds, cashews, walnuts, pistachios, avocados, and fatty fish such as salmon. These foods are excellent sources of unsaturated fats (the good fats) and help to raise your HDL (good) cholesterol.

When using oils (for cooking or for salad dressings), use those with unsaturated fats such as olive oil, corn oil, and other vegetable oils. Stay away from butter, margarine, lard, shortenings, and palm oil.

6. No Soda, No Fruit Juice, and No Dessert

Water, tea, and coffee should be your everyday beverages. In a restaurant setting, order water for your drink. Many people order a soda or dessert in a restaurant under peer pressure. Remember your metabolism has not changed because you are in a restaurant. Sodas contain a significant amount of calories from sugar. Even diet sodas are unhealthy. In my clinical experience, they contribute to a variety of neurological symptoms such as dizziness, headache, and foggy thinking.

Fruit juices contain too much sugar. Instead, have a piece of fresh fruit a day, such as a small apple, pear, apricot, fig, or a few strawberries or blueberries.

Reduce bananas, grapes, watermelon, other melons, mangos, beets, potatoes, and sweet potatoes to special occasions as these can significantly raise your blood sugar. Fruits are a good source for vitamins, but most fruits, especially the sweet ones, are loaded with sugar and usually cause marked elevation in blood sugar in diabetics. Get your vitamins in the form of a pill.

Avoid beer and hard liquor as they cause an increase in blood glucose. A glass of wine two to three times a week is OK.

7. Take a Multi-vitamin

Take a multi-vitamin, chromium picolinate, alpha-lipoic acid, and zinc on a daily basis. See chapter 8 for more information about vitamins and supplements.

8. Say No to Certain Foods

Certain foods cause a marked increase in blood glucose and should be avoided. These foods include pizza, french fries, donuts, pancakes, waffles, fruit juices, and desserts. Leave them for special occasions only.

9. No Buffet, No Fast Food

When you opt for a buffet meal, you want to get the most for your buck (after all, you're only human), and you usually end up overeating.

Most fast foods are loaded with calories and saturated fats. Avoid them.

Try to eat at home as much as possible.

10. Get Involved in Your Food

People often blame someone else, usually a spouse, for their improper meals. Be responsible and get involved in your food. Try to do your own grocery shopping and select healthy food items. Try to prepare your meals yourself as often as you can. It's fun.

Keep a diary of the food you eat and observe the result it has on your blood glucose by checking blood glucose two hours after

Mental Distractions and Eating Do Not Mix

Don't watch TV while eating. Many people overeat because they get too involved in watching a TV show or reading a newspaper and don't keep track of their food intake. Physically you may be sitting at the dining table, but the TV or newspaper takes your mind hundreds and even thousands of miles away. When you're eating, your mind should be *aware* of what you're eating. Taste your meal, chew it properly, enjoy it. Observe other people sitting at the table and the ambience in the room. Relax! Take your time. Don't be in a hurry. Drink plenty of water during your meal.

a meal. Ideally it should be less than 120 mg/dl. Soon you will learn which foods to eat and which ones to avoid. Often, you'll be surprised to see how much you ate, especially when you could have sworn you didn't eat much!

Meal Suggestions

Whether you need to lose weight or simply want to eat in a healthful way, here are some meal suggestions that adhere to my general diet guidelines.

Breakfast Ideas

Cook 1/2 cup of oatmeal in water. Add a handful of crushed nuts. Sprinkle about 1/2 teaspoon of powdered cinnamon.
1 hard-boiled egg (eat egg whites only)
1 cup of 1% milk
1 cup of coffee or tea

Egg-white omelet using 2–3 egg whites only
1 toasted slice of whole wheat bread *without* butter, margarine, jam, jelly, or marmalade
1 cup of coffee or tea or milk

2–4 hard boiled eggs (egg whites only)
1/2 cup of cottage cheese
1 cup of milk
1 cup of coffee or tea

1/2 cup of Cream of Wheat. Add a handful of crushed nuts. Sprinkle about 1/2 teaspoon of powdered cinnamon.
1 cup of milk
1 hard-boiled egg (eat egg whites only)
1 cup of coffee or tea

Lunch/Dinner Ideas

1 cup of coffee or tea
1 bowl of vegetable soup
1 plate of grilled chicken and fresh garden salad (you may add salad dressing)
1 piece of fresh fruit such as a small apple, pear, or plum, or a few strawberries

---

1 cup of coffee or tea
1 bowl of vegetable soup
1 small chicken, turkey, or tuna sandwich. Discard the top slice of bread and make it an open sandwich.
1 piece of fresh fruit such as a small apple, pear, or plum, or a few strawberries

---

Grilled vegetables such as bell pepper, zucchini, or eggplant
Chicken or turkey strips stir-fried
1 glass of wine
1 piece of fresh fruit such as a small apple, pear, or plum, or a
   few strawberries

Steamed vegetables such as broccoli or cauliflower
Grilled chicken or steak
1 small baked potato (without butter or cream)
1 glass of wine
1 piece of fresh fruit such as a small apple, pear, or plum, or a
   few strawberries

Grilled shrimp on a small bed of pasta
1 glass of wine
1 piece of fresh fruit such as a small apple, pear, or plum, or a
   few strawberries

---

1 bowl of soup
Fish, grilled or baked
1 glass of wine
1 piece of fresh fruit such as a small apple, pear, or plum, or a
   few strawberries

6-inch turkey or chicken submarine/deli sandwich. Discard the
   top slice of bread and make it an open sandwich.
A piece of fresh fruit such as a small apple, pear, or plum, or a
   few strawberries

Restaurant/Take-Out Ideas

Chinese

1 cup of wonton soup

Beef, chicken, or shrimp, cooked any Chinese style with a small
portion of steamed rice, such as 1/2 a cup

Hot tea

1 piece of fresh fruit such as a small apple, pear, or plum, or a
few strawberries

Mongolian barbeque beef or chicken

Hot tea

1 piece of fresh fruit such as a small apple, pear, or plum, or a
few strawberries

Japanese

3–4 pieces of sushi. Avoid rolls containing too much rice.

Stir-fried beef or chicken on a small bed of steamed rice such as
1/2 cup

Hot tea

1 piece of fresh fruit such as a small apple, pear, or plum, or a
few strawberries

Mexican

One chicken or beef burrito with beans

Very small amount of rice and guacamole

(no chips or nachos)

1 piece of fresh fruit such as a small apple, pear, or plum, or a
few strawberries

---

1 cup of vegetable soup
1 plate of chicken or beef cooked fajita-style (without the tortillas)
1 cup of beans
1 piece of fresh fruit such as a small apple, pear, or plum, or a few strawberries

---

Indian/Pakistani
Two pieces of tandoori chicken
A small portion of rice, such as 1/2 a cup
Approximately 1 cup of dal
Hot tea
1 piece of fresh fruit such as a small apple, pear, or plum, or a few strawberries

---

Two shish kebabs
1/2 naan
1 plate of vegetables such as okra, spinach, or cauliflower
1 glass of wine
1 piece of fresh fruit such as a small apple, pear, or plum, or a few strawberries

---

1 Samosa
1/2 naan
A small portion of chicken, beef, or lamb curry
Hot tea
1 piece of fresh fruit such as a small apple, pear, or plum, or a few strawberries

Middle Eastern
A small portion of chicken or beef kebab
A small portion of rice, such as 1/2 a cup
1 piece of fresh fruit such as a small apple, pear, or plum, or a
few strawberries

A small portion of chicken shawarma
A small portion of rice, such as 1/2 a cup
1 piece of fresh fruit such as a small apple, pear, or plum, or a
few strawberries

Greek
A small plate of Greek salad
A small portion of gyro meat
(no french fries or rice)
1 piece of fresh fruit such as a small apple, pear, or plum, or a
few strawberries.

If You're a Type 2 Diabetic *and* on Insulin: Diet Guidelines

With the availability of new antidiabetic pills, most Type 2 diabetics should not require insulin. Unfortunately, many are still
treated the old-fashioned way and end up on insulin therapy.

If you are one of these patients, you may be on an insulin pump.
Others use a variety of insulin injections that differ in their onset
and duration of action. On the other hand, only one type of insulin
(either regular insulin or Humalog) is used in an insulin pump.

The Diet for a Type 2 Diabetic Patient on Lantus Once a Day Plus Starlix or Prandin Before Each Meal

Lantus is a newer, long-acting insulin. It provides a steady baseline insulin level for about twenty-four hours. The main advantage of Lantus is that it does not have a peak level as compared to NPH insulin; therefore, patients are at less risk for low blood glucose.

Starlix or Prandin before each meal controls the rise in blood glucose that typically occurs after a meal, even if your premeal blood glucose was normal.

If you are on this regimen, you should eat three small meals a day just like Type 2 diabetics who are not on insulin.

The Diet for a Type 2 Diabetic Patient on Three Insulin Injections per Day

(NPH and Humalog before breakfast, Humalog before lunch, NPH and Humalog before dinner)

NPH starts working in two to three hours, reaches a peak level in about six to eight hours, and has a duration of action of about twelve to sixteen hours.

Humalog is a rapidly acting insulin that starts working within fifteen to thirty minutes; it should therefore be taken just before your meal. Humalog peaks at about one to two hours and duration of action is only three to four hours.

Eat a balanced meal three times per day near the same time every day.

Write down what you eat in a logbook and observe the impact it has on your blood glucose level. Soon you will learn which foods to eat and which foods to avoid.

You will need to adjust your dose of Humalog insulin depending upon the type of meal, your level of blood glucose before the meal, and your level of activity after the meal. Your physicians should provide you with a detailed sliding scale as a guide in order to cover your premeal blood glucose value.

Additional units of Humalog are required to cover the amount of carbohydrates in your meal. As a general rule, 1 unit of Humalog will cover about 10 g of carbohydrates. If you plan an increased level of activity after eating your meal, your dose of Humalog should be decreased.

Talk to you physician—or get recommendations from an endocrinologist—to help you manage your food and insulin intake.

The Diet for a Type 2 Diabetic Patient on the Following Insulin Injections

(NPH and regular insulin before breakfast; regular insulin before lunch; NPH and regular insulin before dinner or regular insulin at dinner and NPH at bedtime)

Remember that NPH starts working in two to three hours, reaches a peak level in about six to eight hours, and has a duration of action of about twelve to sixteen hours. On the other hand, regular insulin starts working in about one hour, reaches a peak in about three to four hours, and has a duration of action of about six to eight hours.

Eat three regular meals and three snacks in between meals: a midmorning snack, a midafternoon snack, and a bedtime snack. Meals and snacks should be about the same time every day.

Write down what you eat in a logbook and observe the impact it has on your blood glucose. Soon you will learn which foods to avoid.

You will need to adjust your dose of regular insulin depending upon the type of meal, your level of blood glucose before the meal, and your level of activity after the meal. Your physician should provide you with a detailed sliding scale as a guide in order to cover your premeal blood glucose value.

Additional units of regular insulin are required to cover the amount of carbohydrates in the meal. As a general rule, 1 unit of regular insulin will cover about 10 g of carbohydrates. If an increased level of activity is planned after the meal, the dose of regular insulin should be decreased.

The Diet for a Type 2 Diabetic Patient on an Insulin Pump

Diabetic patients on an insulin pump have a flexible eating schedule. If you fall into this category, you know that you don't have to eat at a particular time of day.

Patients on an insulin pump have a basal rate of insulin delivery, which helps to control blood glucose levels in the premeal state. In addition, they give a bolus of insulin (Humalog or regular) before each meal to cover for the elevated premeal blood glucose value as well as the anticipated rise in blood glucose after the meal. Your physician should provide a detailed sliding scale, which is your guide to cover your premeal blood glucose value.

Learn how to count the carbohydrates in a meal. Learn to read food labels in the grocery store. As a general rule, 1 unit of Humalog or regular insulin will cover about 10 g of carbohydrates.

Decrease the dose of Humalog or regular insulin if you plan an increased level of activity after the meal such as jogging or biking.

The Myth of Controlling Diabetes with Diet Alone

It is a common misconception among newly diagnosed diabetics that diet alone can control the condition. This is thanks to misleading newspaper and magazine articles oftentimes written by people who don't even treat diabetic patients. Controlling diabetes through diet alone is an old treatment strategy that we now know is ineffective.

In a large clinical trial known as UKPDS (United Kingdom Prospective Diabetes Study), diet alone was compared to drug treatment strategy. Patients in the diet-alone group had higher blood glucose values and suffered from complications of diabetes more frequently than the drug treatment group. Also, diet alone failed to achieve good control of diabetes in more than 80% of patients within one year of the study and these patients had to go on a drug treatment protocol.[1]

Diet is an important part of the treatment of Type 2 diabetes, but it must be used in conjunction with the other four pillars of my treatment strategy.

A common error is that a patient is diagnosed with Type 2 diabetes and instructed to "control it with diet alone." Over the years, I have seen many patients with serious complications of diabetes who were initially told by their physicians to control their diabetes with diet alone. Don't be one of these patients!

CHAPTER 7

Exercise and Managing Your Stress

Exercise is an essential weapon in your arsenal for taking charge of your diabetes. Managing your stress levels—both external and internal—also needs to be an important part of your efforts. Since exercise can help you reduce stress, I've paired these two essential pillars of treatment together in this chapter.

You've likely been told before that exercise is important. But did you know that exercise reduces insulin resistance? Therefore, it not only helps to reduce your blood glucose levels but also to prevent deadly complications of diabetes.

Everyone knows that exercise is good for your health, but most people don't put that knowledge into regular action. There is a good chance that you own a treadmill that is collecting dust in your garage or you're a member of a gym that you haven't visited in months. Why? If you look at it logically, you'll realize that you like the concept of exercise more than exercising itself.

As long as you don't have a membership to a gym or you don't have the right machine at home, you have the perfect excuse for not exercising. Then one day, you purchase a membership or a machine. Soon the thrill of shopping is over and so is the whole idea of exercising. Now your excuse is that you don't have time to go to the gym or you're too tired to get on the machine at home!

Once you fully understand your superficial and emotional attachment to the concept of exercise, wake up and get serious about exercise itself. Realize that you can start exercising right *now* without any memberships or expensive machines. Do some exercise now!

Take a break from reading this book and exercise. Don't postpone it until you can fit it into your busy schedule. That day will never come. Until you make your exercise routine a high priority, you will always be too busy doing something else.

I'm not suggesting that you have to set your sights on running a marathon or that you should start training for a triathlon! I'm not even suggesting that you have to regularly do aerobics or weight training at your gym. Any manner of exercise will be helpful, will help you relax (reduce stress), and will ultimately help reduce your insulin resistance. Adding any amount of exercise to your life—now—will be beneficial.

Simple walking for about thirty minutes every day is a good exercise program. Actually, it's a better exercise program for diabetics than a treadmill and other similar machines. The reason is that by the time they are diagnosed with diabetes, most diabetics have developed some damage to the long nerves in their legs. The impact of running on a treadmill or jogging can cause more damage to these nerves.

Many diabetic patients have also developed some eye damage due to uncontrolled diabetes. Often patients, especially those older than sixty years old, have developed some degenerative arthritis in their knees or hips. Jogging and running can further worsen their eye disease and degenerative arthritis. Even middle-aged people are at risk for developing arthritis if they use their joints too vigorously, as is often the case in regular gym-goers. Remember, insulin resistance (and therefore, diabetes) is likely to worsen as you age, and you're going to need your legs to exercise, especially in your golden years.

In addition to regular walking, try parking your car in the far corner of the parking lot to get that extra few minutes of walking. As an added bonus, you'll avoid the stress of finding the perfect parking spot right in front of the store. Try taking the stairs for a couple of flights instead of elevators or escalators. Walk in the mall, in the grocery store, at the outlet mall, and downtown.

Go to a nearby park every day. When I walk in my neighborhood park in the evening, I'm often the only one there. It's sad. I wonder where everyone is. There is a beautiful park five minutes from my clinic that I often visit during lunchtime. I mentioned it to one of my patients who complained about not having a treadmill at home as an excuse for not exercising. On his next visit, he still had not been to this park and was still waiting for his daughter to buy him a treadmill.

In the greater Los Angeles area there are three large, beautiful gardens open to the public. I often ask my patients if they have visited any of these gardens. They look at me with surprise. Most of them haven't even heard about these great places. Spending some time in public parks and gardens is a great way to exercise. It's also wonderful for reducing stress.

I find *yoga* to be a good exercise for all age groups. It is joint friendly, and certain yoga postures can actually help with arthritis pain. Start out slowly. Do what you can easily do and, like any other exercise program, gradually build it up. Find a yoga class in your neighborhood. Yoga—and the meditative state that it helps you achieve—will also help you deal with everyday stress.

Swimming is also a good alternative for diabetics with peripheral nerve disease, eye disease, and/or arthritis.

You should consult your physician before beginning an exercise plan. As a general rule, exercise should be started at a low level and duration and intensity should be increased gradually. If you have heart disease or suspect you may have heart disease, check with your cardiologist before starting an exercise program.

Vigorous exercise can lower blood glucose too much, especially if you're on drugs such as Prandin, Starlix, insulin, or sulfonylurea drugs (including those such as Glucotrol, Amaryl, Glynase, glipizide, glyburide). Therefore, always carry candy while exercising. (Newer antidiabetic drugs such as Actos, Avandia, and metformin do not cause low blood sugar by themselves because they do not increase your insulin production.)

Also, check your blood sugar before starting your exercise routine. If your blood sugar is below 100 mg/dl, eat something before you begin. Also, check your blood sugar at the end of your exercise.

Managing Stress

Sometimes your blood glucose goes up without any obvious reason. No change in diet, no change in exercise routine, no change in medicine, no illness. You wonder what happened. What increased your blood glucose? Often, the culprit is stress.

How Stress Affects a Diabetic Person

You may have heard of the "mind-body connection" and it's real: the mind is intimately connected to the rest of the body through a web of nerves and hormones.

A stressed-out mind affects your body in a number of ways:

- It increases the production of two hormones: cortisol and catecholamine from the adrenal glands
- It also stimulates a special network of nerves in the body, known as the autonomic nervous system

Both of these changes worsen your insulin resistance, which in turn results in an increase in blood glucose, as well as an increase in blood pressure.

Normally, cortisol has what is called a diurnal rhythm: it is at its maximum level early in the morning and then gradually declines as the day progresses, reaching its lowest point around midnight. There is good reason for this: cortisol increases glucose production by the liver early in the morning, supplying the body with fuel in preparation for the day. In the evening, cortisol levels drop significantly, which helps you wind down and fall asleep.

Stress wrecks havoc with your biological clock. It causes your cortisol to be elevated all the time and, in turn, increases your blood glucose level as well as your blood pressure. It's no wonder that when you are feeling anxious or under pressure you might have trouble sleeping, and you might feel as though you have an excess of anxiety or anxious energy.

Stress also affects the autonomic nervous system. In a diabetic person, the autonomic nervous system is under attack from two fronts: one from diabetes itself and the other from stress. Many complications of diabetes develop through autonomic neuropathy. Some manifestations of diabetic autonomic neuropathy include stomach bloating, diarrhea, constipation, urinary frequency, and impotence. (For details see the section on nerve disease in chapter 11.)

Stress also decreases your intellectual functioning and causes memory loss.

The Two Types of Stress

I categorize stress into two types: external stress and internal stress. External stress is the stress we are all familiar with: you lose your job, your mom is in the hospital, your brother-in-law wrecks your car. External stress is brought about by your experience of events that are outside your control. Still, there are things you can usually do—actions you can take—to help you deal with the external events that cause you stress: you can look for a new job, talk to your mother's doctor about her prognosis, and have your car fixed—on your brother-in-law's dime! In terms of taking charge of your stress in order to take charge of your diabetes, it's important to look carefully at your life and try to eliminate sources of external stress when possible. If your job causes you great stress, it might be time to consider a career—or at least a company—change. If sitting in endless traffic during your commute makes you anxious, look for alternatives, including carpooling, public transportation, or even negotiating a different start time (flex hours).

And then there is internal stress. Internal stress comes from the memory of psychological events in your life, often buried deep in your psyche but very much alive and very powerful. Internal stress might feel like background noise, a nagging voice, the ever-busy mind that keeps your mind restless even when you are trying to relax on a beach in Hawaii. In a lot of ways, internal stress is the harder of the two types to deal with because we are often unaware that we are experiencing internal stress and its causes are mostly unexamined. Moreover, a person with unexamined internal stress reacts strongly to external stressful situations and thus increases his or her stress level several-fold.

Your psychosocial conditioning from childhood plays a major role in creating this internal stress. This conditioned mind either keeps you in the past or takes you into the future, bypassing the reality of the present moment. Therefore, psychologically speaking, you either live under long shadows of the past, trying to deal with undesirable, painful events, or your busy mind takes you into the future, creating fear and worries that may never come to pass. Now *logically* speaking, the past is gone and the future never arrives; the past is history and the future is an illusion, a fantasy, a virtual world. But your psychological busy mind is *illogical*. It is constantly avoiding the present moment, the only real moment in your life. Physically, you are in the present moment, but psychologically, you are miles or years away, lost in the past or worrying about the future. This conflict between mind and body is the basis of internal stress. Your body doesn't like it.

For example, you're driving on the freeway, but your busy mind is thinking about the bitter argument you had with your wife over the weekend—"We can barely pay the mortgage and she's buying $200 shoes like money grows on trees!"—and the next moment, you're thinking about your upcoming doctor appointment—"Maybe he'll tell me I have cancer, and then I'll probably die a miserable death in a year, nauseated the whole time from chemotherapy just like my Uncle Bob." Physically, you are on the freeway, but mentally you are far away, lost in the past and worrying about the future. It is this division of your body being in the present and your mind being in the past or future that creates internal conflict and internal stress. Your ever-busy mind, working like a compulsive noise machine, is the root cause of your internal stress.

And it's not only our personal memories, worries, or unhappiness that creates internal stress. Most of us start out our day by turning on the TV, reading the newspaper, checking our e-mail, and noting Wall Street's performance along with the news on the Internet. We share any sensational news that happened thousands of miles away with our coworkers and then together we worry about our future and so on and so on. We avoid the present moment and instead we often talk about what we did last weekend or what we are going to do next month. We are all so immersed in this behavior that it seems perfectly normal, so real—but actually it is not. Mostly we live in the virtual world.

Getting Rid of Internal Stress

Your ever-busy chattering mind, the root cause of your internal stress, needs to calm down. How? Not by trying to fight, control, or suppress it. That only makes matters worse. Your busy mind loves to hide in the past or in the future. It avoids the present moment and does not like to be looked at. It loves when you are on autopilot, totally unaware. So instead, use wisdom and be observant. Each time you see that your busy mind has wandered to the past or the future, gently bring it back to the present moment. Living in the present moment is the key to eliminating internal stress and discovering your own inner peace and joy.

Keep your mind where your body is. For example, while driving on the freeway, keep your mind on the drive. Notice the variety of cars and trucks, the budding leaves on passing trees, and the moving clouds in the sky. You may pass this route hundreds of times, but if you *really* look, you will see new things every day.

While waiting in the exam room for your doctor to arrive, keep your mind in the present by observing everything in the room—an acrylic sculpture of the heart, a painting of a field of flowers, or the plaid curtains on the window. Be aware of your busy mind that often creeps in and starts interpreting or judging. "Those plaid curtains are hideous. I would have chosen something like the blue ones in my guest room." And you start thinking about all the problems you had installing the curtains in your house. Now your mind is in control again and you are *gone* from the present moment. Maybe the acrylic heart sculpture reminds you that you may have a heart attack one day, and, suddenly, you are imagining how your spouse will react as the ER technicians try to revive you as you lie dying on the green carpet in your bedroom. POOF! See how easily we disappear from the present by small distractions?

Just be present without interpretations or judgments. Every now and then, pay attention to your breathing, which will immediately bring you to the present moment. As soon as you are in the present moment, your internal stress dissipates and your inner peace and joy will have an opportunity to shine through. Initially, you may be fully aware of being in the present moment for just a few seconds, but gradually your busy mind will start to calm down and you'll be able to stay in the present moment for longer periods of time. You will be surprised at the immense reservoir of joy and peace right there inside of you that you were so unaware of before. This is your true self. Once you have discovered your true self, you will also be able to face external stress in a much better way. For example, in a traffic jam, you will observe so many details that you otherwise would have missed. Psychologically speaking, you will gradually learn to be free from your internal as well as external stress.

CHAPTER 8

Vitamins and Herbal Medicines

Vitamins and herbal medicines have been extensively used in the treatment of diabetes. However, because some practitioners of alternative medicine have made exuberant and sometimes irresponsible claims about the efficacy of vitamins and herbs, most mainstream physicians in the U.S. totally ignore these valuable and helpful agents.

I have reviewed published data about vitamins and herbs and take a middle-of-the road approach.

By themselves, vitamins and herbs may not provide adequate treatment, but they are certainly helpful as an adjunctive therapy. Published data as well as my own extensive clinical experience on the following vitamins and herbs appear to indicate that they reduce insulin resistance. Therefore, I recommend them as an adjunctive therapy for my diabetic patients.

- Alpha-lipoic acid
- Chromium picolinate
- Fenugreek
- Nopal

My Clinical Experience with Vitamins and Herbs

In the last five years I have extensively used alpha-lipoic acid, chromium picolinate, cinnamon, coenzyme Q10, magnesium, and vitamin B12 in my diabetic patients and have found these supplements to be beneficial and safe. Alpha-lipoic acid is especially helpful in patients with peripheral neuropathy. Vitamin B12 in high doses is helpful for fatigue, peripheral neuropathy, and, in combination with high doses of folic acid, helps lower homocysteine levels, which reduces the risk for heart disease and strokes.

Safety

I routinely check liver and kidney function, cholesterol panel, and blood counts in my diabetic patients. I have found no adverse effects of herbal medication on the liver, kidney, cholesterol, or blood count. Also, my patients are frequently on medicines to treat diabetes, blood pressure, cholesterol, coronary artery disease, and thyroid disorders and are on multiple medications. I have found no clinical adverse interactions between vitamins and medications.

However, it is possible that any of these vitamins/herbs may interact with other medicines that you take. For example, any of these vitamins/herbs may have additive effects to insulin or oral antidiabetic medications that results in low blood glucose levels. Therefore, it is important that you check with your physician or other health care provider before you go on any of these vitamins/herbs. In general, these vitamins/herbs have not been tested in pregnant and nursing mothers, and therefore should be avoided by them.

- Cinnamon
- Coenzyme Q10
- Magnesium
- Vitamin B12

Alpha-lipoic Acid

Alpha-lipoic acid is normally produced in small quantities in our cells and helps in the normal metabolism of glucose. In pharmacologic doses, it functions as a strong antioxidant. Alpha-lipoic acid also regenerates other antioxidants including vitamin C, vitamin E, and coenzyme Q10. Cells of diabetic patients are under a tremendous amount of oxidative stress, which is why it makes perfect sense to use alpha-lipoic acid in diabetics as a supplement.

Based upon a number of scientific studies[1] and my own extensive clinical experience, it's clear to me that alpha-lipoic acid decreases insulin resistance and promotes healthy nerve function.

This product has been used in Germany for more than thirty years in the treatment of diabetic neuropathy. In Germany, fifteen clinical trials on alpha-lipoic acid have been completed and have shown the effectiveness of alpha-lipoic acid in treating peripheral as well as cardiac autonomic neuropathy.[2] (See chapter 11 to learn more about diabetic neuropathy.)

Sources

Alpha-lipoic acid is found in beef, kidney, heart, broccoli, spinach, and yeast. However, the quantity of alpha-lipoic acid from food sources is small. Therefore, it needs to be taken as a supplement in the form of pills.

Recommended Dose

The usual dose that I use in my patients is 600–1200 mg/day. Doses up to 1800 mg/day have been used in clinical trials without any significant side effects. Doses under 600 mg/day are not effective for nerve health.

You can get alpha-lipoic acid in drug, health food, and vitamin stores as well as on the Internet. Alpha-lipoic acid is also included in multivitamins for diabetic patients. However, my research has found that in most multivitamins, the quantities of alpha-lipoic acid are too small, such as 100 mg. If you buy it individually, it is usually available in 100 mg, 200 mg, 300 mg, and 600 mg capsules. Remember, you need to take a daily dose of at least 600 mg to see its beneficial effects.

Safety

Alpha-lipoic acid has been found to be safe in clinical use. In my extensive clinical experience, I have found a handful of people with GERD (gastroesophageal reflux disease, also known as hiatal hernia) who experience worsening of their heartburn on alpha-lipoic acid, which subsides after stopping the supplement. Also, thiamine (vitamin B1) deficiency may be aggravated by alpha-lipoic acid. Therefore, any person at risk for thiamine deficiency, particularly alcoholics, should also take thiamine if they decide to take alpha-lipoic acid. Thiamine is found in most multivitamins. As alpha-lipoic acid may help to lower blood glucose, diabetics on insulin and oral antidiabetic drugs may potentially experience abnormally low blood glucose levels (hypoglycemia). Close monitoring of blood glucose is important. You should also let your physician know if you decide to take alpha-lipoic acid or any supplement. There is no safety data on alpha-lipoic acid regarding pregnancy or lactation. Therefore, alpha-lipoic acid should be avoided by pregnant and nursing women.

Caution

People with GERD (hiatal hernia), or any other stomach ailments should take alpha-lipoic acid supplements with caution.

Chromium Picolinate

Chromium is required for the normal metabolism of glucose, and it enhances the effects of insulin in our body. Because resistance to the action of insulin (insulin resistance) is the hallmark of impaired glucose tolerance (prediabetes) and Type 2 diabetes, it makes sense to use chromium in these individuals. Additionally, Type 2 diabetics have been found to have an increased loss of chromium through their urine.

Several studies have shown the beneficial effects of chromium supplementation in diabetic patients. The results of an excellent placebo-controlled study conducted in China showed that chromium picolinate might be beneficial in the treatment of Type 2 diabetes. In this study, 180 patients with Type 2 diabetes were randomly divided into three groups and supplemented with either a placebo, 200 mcg/day, or 1000 mcg/day of chromium picolinate. The results showed that glycated hemoglobin (a measure of long-term glucose control) as well as insulin levels were significantly lower in both chromium picolinate treatment groups when compared to the placebo group.[3]

Sources

Chromium is naturally found in small amounts in foods such as whole grains, processed meats, broccoli, green beans, cheese, and brewer's yeast.

Recommended Dose

The usual dose that I use in my patients is 200 mcg/day. It is readily available wherever vitamins are sold.

Safety

Several studies have shown chromium intake of up to 1000 mcg per day to be safe. My own extensive clinical experience testifies to this. However, there have been isolated reports of serious side effects due to chromium picolinate.

In one case, kidney and liver dysfunction developed after taking 1200–2400 mcg/day of chromium for five months for weight loss. In another case, kidney failure was reported in a twenty-four-year-old who took a supplement containing chromium picolinate for two weeks during workout sessions. I do not recommend chromium picolinate supplements for weight loss or building muscle.

Fenugreek

Fenugreek is an herb that has been used in India for ages in the treatment of diabetes. Several clinical trials carried out in India have shown that fenugreek seeds can lower blood glucose levels in diabetic patients.

An excellent clinical trial demonstrated that fenugreek treatment not only lowered glucose levels but also reduced insulin resistance, lowered serum triglycerides level, and increased HDL cholesterol levels in Type 2 diabetic patients. No side effects were reported.[4]

Recommended Dose

The recommended dose of fenugreek has not yet been established. The typical range is from 5 to 30 g of fenugreek seed powder with each meal. You can buy fenugreek seed powder where a large variety of herbs are sold, including many health food stores as well as on the Internet. Indian grocery stores are a particularly good place to find fenugreek seed powder at a low cost.

Caution

Fenugreek may interfere with clotting. Therefore, patients on chronic Coumadin (warfarin) therapy should avoid this supplement.

Nopal

Nopal (Opuntia streptacantha), or the prickly pear cactus, has been used for glucose control in Mexico for centuries. Studies have reported improvement in glucose control and a decrease in insulin levels indicating a decrease in insulin resistance with the use of nopal.[5] No side effects have been reported.

Recommended Dose

The recommended dose of nopal has not yet been established. One can eat one half of a prickly pear a day, eating the flesh and discarding the seeds. Many people find it is pleasant to eat nopal chopped up and sprinkled in a salad. You can find nopal (prickly pear) in Mexican grocery markets. Some health food stores also carry nopal.

Cinnamon

Physicians have long been intrigued by the beneficial effects of cinnamon. In December 2003, an excellent study was published in *Diabetes Care*. In this study, investigators from Pakistan used cinnamon powder in sixty patients with Type 2 diabetes. Three daily doses were used: 1 g, 3 g, and 6 g. The researchers found a decrease of 18%–29% in blood glucose in these patients. Their serum triglycerides also decreased by 23%–30%. Patients consuming 6 g of cinnamon powder appeared to have achieved results earlier, but by forty days, all doses had the same efficacy.[6]

Recommended Dose

You can use one teaspoonful of cinnamon powder three times a day. You can sprinkle it over cereal, oatmeal, Cream of Wheat, tea, or coffee. Cinnamon is easily available in the form of a powder from grocery stores. It is also available in pill form in some health food and vitamin stores as well as over the Internet.

Coenzyme Q10 (CoQ10)

Coenzyme Q10 is a strong antioxidant. It is found in a large variety of plants and animals, but for medical purposes, it is easily available in the form of tablets and capsules. Coenzyme Q10 improves diastolic dysfunction of the heart in patients with hypertension, which is commonly present in patients with diabetes. It has also been shown to lower blood glucose levels.

Recommended Dose

Though there is no recommended established dose for coenzyme Q10, the usual dose varies from 20 mg to 150 mg/day. Coenzyme Q10 can be bought in tablet or capsule form.

Note

Statin drugs such as simvastatin (Zocor), atorvastatin (Lipitor), and pravastatin (Pravachol) are commonly used in diabetic patients. These are excellent drugs that lower LDL cholesterol very effectively. Unfortunately, these drugs can also lower the level of CoQ10 as demonstrated in a study at Columbia University in New York.[7] This may explain the muscle aches that patients often complain of while on a statin drug.

Magnesium

Magnesium is a mineral and an important component of a healthy diet. It helps the function of muscles, nerves, and the heart. It also plays an important role in the metabolism of glucose. In one study, magnesium deficiency produced insulin resistance in otherwise healthy people.[8] Several studies have shown magnesium supplementation to be beneficial for Type 2 diabetic patients.

Sources

Dietary sources of magnesium include nuts, seeds, fish, oysters, scallops, beans, lentils, milk, yogurt, broccoli, okra, spinach, artichokes, and whole grain bread.

Recommended Dose

The Recommended Daily Allowance (RDA) of magnesium is 400 mg/day. Magnesium is available in pill form. Many multivitamins include magnesium.

Caution

Patients with kidney failure should be very careful about magnesium intake as these individuals can develop a high level of magnesium in their blood that can be life threatening. Therefore, anyone with kidney problems should follow their physician's recommendation about magnesium intake.

Vitamin B12

Vitamin B12 is one of the most important vitamins in our body. It helps repair DNA in every cell of the body and is important in maintaining the integrity of our genome.

Vitamin B12 is particularly important for the health of the brain, nerves, blood cells, fatty acid metabolism, the gastrointestinal tract, and the heart. It becomes especially important for the health of diabetics who are already at a high risk for peripheral nerve disease, autonomic nerve disease, heart disease, and memory loss. Metformin, a drug used by many diabetics, often lowers vitamin B12 levels.

Sources

Animal products are the main natural sources of vitamin B12. Plant-derived food is devoid of vitamin B12. Good dietary sources include egg yolks, salmon, crabs, oysters, clams, sardines, liver, brain, and kidney. Smaller amounts of vitamin B12 are also found in beef, lamb, chicken, pork, milk, and cheese.

The Impact of Low Vitamin B12

- Lack of energy
- Tingling and numbness in the feet and hands due to peripheral neuropathy
- Memory loss, dementia, and depression
- Abnormal gait and lack of balance
- Increase in the level of homocysteine, which is a risk factor for heart disease and stroke; low folic acid is the other contributory factor for raising homocysteine levels
- Burning of the tongue, poor appetite, constipation alternating with diarrhea, vague abdominal pain
- Anemia

Those at Risk for Low Vitamin B12

- Anyone on metformin (Glucophage, Fortamet, Glumetza), a drug commonly prescribed for diabetics
- Anyone on a strict vegetarian diet, because vegetables are devoid of vitamin B12

ı stomach medicines such as Prilosec, Prevacid,
Aciphex, Pepcid, Zantac, Tagamet, etc.
aking antibiotics, which can lower vitamin B12 by
ıg with normal intestinal bacterial flora
- Anyone who has undergone stomach surgery
- Anyone with gastrointestinal disorders such as chronic pancreatitis, atrophic gastritis, small intestinal resection or bypass, gluten enteropathy, Crohn's disease, and malignancy

Diagnosing Vitamin B12 Deficiency

Vitamin B12 deficiency often remains undiagnosed because physicians generally don't think of it as a possibility. For example, when a diabetic patient complains of tingling in their feet, physicians do all the workup to diagnose diabetic peripheral neuropathy. They then start you on a drug treatment, often without checking your vitamin B12 level, even if you are on metformin.

In reality, peripheral neuropathy in diabetic patients on metformin is often due to two factors: diabetes itself and vitamin B12 deficiency.

Vitamin B12 deficiency can be diagnosed by a blood test. A blood level that is lower than 400 pg/ml indicates vitamin B12 deficiency. In my clinical experience, patients do much better when their vitamin B12 level is close to 1000 pg/ml.

Recommended Dose

The amount of vitamin B12 present in the typical multivitamin is often not enough to meet the special needs of diabetic patients, especially when they are also on the medications listed above.

Vitamin B12 supplements are available as oral pills and as pills for sublingual absorption (under the tongue). I prefer the sublingual absorption route because the absorption of vitamin B12 from the oral cavity (as it dissolves in the mouth) is better than absorption from the stomach and intestines.

Vitamin B12 is also available in the form of an injection. You need a prescription from a physician for a vitamin B12 injection.

To my knowledge, there are no reported cases of vitamin B12 overdoses in medical literature. Vitamin B12 in high doses along with folic acid and vitamin B6 helps to lower homocysteine level, and thus helps lower the risk for heart disease and strokes.

Glupride Multi

Glupride Multi is a daily multivitamin I created for the special needs of diabetics. As you now must realize, diabetics greatly benefit from taking these vitamins and herbs, but they must take them in the correct amounts to reap the benefits. In response to these real-life challenges, I formulated Glupride Multi.

Glupride Multi contains twenty-one vitamins/herbs including alpha-lipoic acid, chromium picolinate, coenzyme Q10, magnesium, cinnamon, and vitamin B12. In addition, Glupride Multi also contains vitamins A, B complex, C, E, folic acid, zinc, selenium, iodine, and vanadium.

I specifically excluded potassium, vitamin K, iron, and calcium (which are contained in most multivitamins) from Glupride Multi.

I excluded potassium for the following reason. Most diabetic patients have some degree of kidney dysfunction. Many are also on drugs called ACE inhibitors or ARB drugs. (See page 199 for a list of ACE inhibitors and ARB drugs.) These drugs can potentially increase blood potassium levels, especially in the presence of kidney disease. A high level of potassium in the blood can be life threatening. These patients certainly do not need extra potassium in their multivitamin.

I excluded vitamin K for the following reason. Insulin resistance is the root cause of diabetes in most diabetic patients. For this reason, they are at an increased risk for clot formation, which is the cause of most heart attacks and strokes. Vitamin K can potentially further increase already elevated levels of "clotting factors" in the blood of those individuals with insulin resistance. Also, some diabetic patients also take a blood thinner called Coumadin (warfarin). Vitamin K can potentially interfere with the efficacy of Coumadin, creating a serious health problem.

I excluded iron and calcium for the following reason. Many diabetic patients are also on thyroid hormones such as levothyroxine. Iron and calcium, if taken at the same time as a thyroid hormone, can interfere with the absorption of the thyroid hormone. Iron and calcium should be taken at least three hours apart from a thyroid hormone.

Glupride Multi is available for purchase from my website, www.onlinemedinfo.com or you can call 1-888-495-2002.

CHAPTER 9

Using Prescription Medications to Help Control Type 2 Diabetes

Now we come to what I see as the fifth important pillar of treatment, or the fifth weapon in our arsenal to manage Type 2 diabetes: prescription drugs. As you know, most doctors use a step-up approach to diabetes medications. That is, they keep increasing the dosage and number of medications to treat your diabetes.

In contrast, and as alluded to earlier in this book, I have achieved excellent results with a step-down approach to using drugs in the treatment of diabetes. I focus on treating Insulin Resistance—the root cause of diabetes—first and foremost. My clinical experience bears this out. The detailed case studies in this chapter are included to help you understand how I prescribe medications in my practice. In taking charge of your own diabetes, and in talking with your specialist about incorporating my treatment recommendations, you might find these case studies an effective way to start that important conversation.

A good way to begin the discussion of the use of antidiabetic medications to treat Type 2 diabetes is to review the medications currently available in the U.S.

Here is a listing of all the currently available antidiabetic medications listed by their brand as well as generic names, followed by more detailed and specific information about their use (organized by the class of drug). Later, I explain in detail how I utilize these drugs to manage diabetes in my patients.

Brand Name	Generic Name	Mechanism of Action	Class of Drugs
Actos	Pioglitazone	Primarily treats insulin resistance at the level of muscle and fat cells	Thiazolidinediones (TZD)
Avandia	Rosiglitazone		
Glucophage Fortamet Glumetza Riomet	Metformin	Primarily treats insulin resistance at the level of the liver	Biguanides
Amaryl	Glimepiride	Increases insulin production	Sulfonylurea agents
Diabeta Micronase Glynase	Glyburide		
Glucotrol	Glipizide		
Diabinese	Chlorpropamide		
Prandin	Repaglinide	Increases insulin production	Meglitinides
Starlix	Nateglinide	Increases insulin production	Amino acid derivatives
Precose	Acarbose	Decreases glucose absorption from the intestine after a meal	Alpha-glucosidase inhibitors
Glyset	Miglitol		

(continues)

Brand Name	Generic Name	Mechanism of Action	Class of Drugs
Byetta	Exenatide	Increases insulin production, decreases glucagon* secretion, reduces stomach emptying, and decreases appetite	Incretin mimetic agent
Januvia	Sitagliptin	Increases insulin production, decreases glucagon secretion	DPP-4 inhibitor; increases naturally occurring incretin hormones in the body

Combination Drugs

Brand Name	Generic Name
Actoplus met	Combination of pioglitazone and metformin
Avandamet	Combination of rosiglitazone and metformin
Glucovance	Combination of metformin & glyburide
Duetact	Combination of pioglitazone & glimepiride
Avandaryl	Combination of rosiglitazone & glimepiride

*Glucagon is a hormone produced by the alpha cells of the pancreas. It increases blood glucose.

Medications Used to
Treat Type 2 Diabetics in the U.S.

Various types of insulin are still being used to treat Type 2 diabetes. For a detailed description of insulin types, please refer to pages 150–151.

Actos (generic: pioglitazone),
Avandia (generic: rosiglitazone)

Actos (pioglitazone) and Avandia (rosiglitazone) belong to the relatively newer class of drugs known as TZD (short for thiazolidinedione) drugs. They were released in the U.S. in 1999. Actos (pioglitazone) and Avandia (rosiglitazone) are similar drugs. You may be prescribed one or the other, but not both.

Actos (pioglitazone) and Avandia (rosiglitazone) treat insulin resistance at the level of muscles and fat, which are the two most important sites where insulin resistance takes place. These drugs also modestly reduce insulin resistance in the liver, which is the third site of insulin resistance. As a result of reduction in insulin resistance, your body's own insulin becomes more efficient in lowering blood glucose.

Actos (pioglitazone) and Avandia (rosiglitazone) have a slow onset of action. You do not see any significant effect on blood glucose during the first two weeks of therapy. You will see their peak effect at three to four months of therapy.

Advantages

- While on Actos (pioglitazone) and Avandia (rosiglitazone), you don't need to worry about low blood glucose
- Unlike older drugs such as glyburide or glipizide, Actos (pioglitazone) and Avandia (rosiglitazone) don't stress the in-

sulin producing cells (beta cells) of the pancreas. Therefore, you continue to have good control of diabetes for a long period of time and don't end up on insulin, which is usually what happens if you are on drugs such as glyburide or glipizide without the addition of Actos or Avandia.

- In addition to controlling blood glucose, Actos (pioglitazone) and Avandia (rosiglitazone) have other beneficial effects. They lower serum triglycerides and raise HDL (good) cholesterol. A good level of HDL cholesterol is the most important factor that reduces your risk for heart attack, stroke, dementia, and leg amputation.

- Narrowing of the blood vessels (also known as atherosclerosis) is very common in diabetic patients. That is why you are at a very high risk for heart attack, stroke, dementia, and leg amputation. Actos (pioglitazone) and Avandia (rosiglitazone) can reduce this narrowing of the blood vessels. This extraordinary effect is unique to these drugs. In an excellent study published in 2001 in the *Journal of Clinical Endocrinology and Metabolism* researchers were able to show a reduction in the thickness of the carotid artery wall in diabetic patients treated with pioglitazone (Actos).[1]

- Diabetic patients have a high level of a substance called PAI-1 (plasminogen activator inhibitor-1). This abnormality places you at high risk for clot formation and an increased risk for clot-related events such as a heart attack and stroke. Actos (pioglitazone) and Avandia (rosiglitazone) decrease the level of PAI-1 and therefore can prevent heart attack and stroke.

- Diabetics who undergo balloon angioplasty of narrowed coronary arteries frequently develop another blockage after just a few months. This occurs due to the formation of a new layer of lining of the blood vessel wall, known as neointima formation. Actos (pioglitazone) and Avandia (rosiglitazone) have been shown to reduce neointima formation. Thus, these drugs can reduce the need for repeated angioplasties.[2]

Disadvantages

- While on Actos (pioglitazone) or Avandia (rosiglitazone) you may experience some weight gain and ankle swelling. This happens primarily due to retention of water. If you already have congestive heart failure (weak heart), these medications can be problematic, as these can worsen your heart failure. These drugs can cause congestive heart failure even if you did not have it before. Therefore, while on these drugs, you should watch out for any signs of congestive heart failure, which include shortness of breath, ankle swelling, and excessive weight gain without any excess in food intake.

- You may also see a mild elevation in LDL cholesterol, which may appear as an undesirable effect, but in fact, is not. The explanation for this phenomenon is as follows. LDL cholesterol has two subpopulations: small, dense LDL particles (which are more harmful) and large, fluffy particles (which are less harmful). Actos (pioglitazone) and Avandia (rosiglitazone) cause a shift from the small, dense particles to the large, fluffy particles. As the size of LDL cholesterol particle increases, the total quantity of LDL cholesterol rises. However, this transformed, "fluffy" LDL cholesterol is less dangerous. Actos (pioglitazone) and Avandia (rosiglitazone) also increase HDL cholesterol. The ratio of HDL to LDL cholesterol essentially remains unchanged or may even improve.

Caution

Actos (pioglitazone) or Avandia (rosiglitazone) should not be used if you have any degree of congestive heart failure.

Glucophage, Fortamet, Glumetza, Riomet
(generic: metformin)

Metformin was released for use in the U.S. in 1994 under the brand name of Glucophage, although it had been in use in other parts of the world for many years. Now metformin is also available under several other brand names such as Fortamet, Glumetza, and Riomet, as well as in its generic name. Riomet is unique in that it is available as a liquid.

Metformin primarily acts by reducing insulin resistance at the level of the liver. Normally, the liver is actively producing glucose during the night when you are asleep. In Type 2 diabetic patients, this phenomenon is exaggerated. Now you understand why you may wake up with high blood glucose even though you didn't eat anything overnight. Metformin reduces this excess glucose production by the liver and helps to lower your morning blood glucose.

Advantages

- Metformin by itself does not cause low blood glucose
- Metformin modestly reduces serum triglycerides
- Metformin also causes some weight loss

Disadvantages

- Nausea, abdominal upset, and diarrhea are fairly common side effects due to metformin. If you experience any of these symptoms, either reduce the dose or even stop the drug completely, but only after checking with your physician.
- Sometimes patients report a metallic taste in their mouths, which curbs a person's appetite. This side effect may work to your advantage by helping you lose weight.
- Deficiency of vitamin B12 can also develop. In my experience, this is a common side effect. Vitamin B12 deficiency

can cause tingling and numbness in the feet and hands (peripheral neuropathy), forgetfulness (dementia), low blood count (anemia), and an increase in homocysteine levels, which is a risk factor for heart disease and stroke. Therefore, it is a good idea to check your vitamin B12 level in a blood test. If the level is low or in the low–normal range, start taking vitamin B12. Alternately, you can start taking vitamin B12 if you are on metformin, even without checking your blood level of vitamin B12. You don't need to worry about too much vitamin B12 as there are no reported cases of vitamin B12 overdose.

- A serious but rare side effect of metformin is lactic acidosis, a condition diagnosed on blood testing. This can occur if metformin is used in patients with kidney failure, liver disease, heart failure, emphysema, or shock. Lactic acidosis carries a high mortality rate. Therefore, metformin should not be used in the above-mentioned conditions.

Caution

- Metformin should not be used if you have liver dysfunction, kidney failure, heart failure, or an acute illness
- You should withhold metformin for twenty-four hours after a procedure involving administration of a dye, such as a coronary angiogram or CT scan. The rational for this precaution is that you may develop kidney failure after these types of procedures. If metformin is continued in the presence of kidney failure, you can develop lactic acidosis. A blood test for kidney function (serum creatinine) should be performed twenty-four hours after the procedure. You can resume metformin if this test is normal.

Amaryl (generic: glimepiride), Micronase
(generic: glyburide), Diabeta (generic: glyburide),
Glynase (generic: glyburide), Glucotrol (generic: glipizide),
Diabinese (generic: chlorpropamide)

These drugs are called sulfonylurea drugs. Before 1994, these were the only oral drugs available in the U.S. for the treatment of Type 2 diabetes. These drugs stimulate the pancreas to produce more insulin. Their effect usually lasts for about twenty-four hours. In patients with kidney failure, their effect can last up to two to three days.

Advantages

These drugs start working immediately and are very effective in lowering blood glucose in the short term

Disadvantages

- These drugs do not treat insulin resistance, the underlying disease process of diabetics
- While on these drugs your blood glucose can drop too low (hypoglycemia). Symptoms of low blood sugar include palpitations of the heart, excessive sweating, weakness, dizziness, a feeling of passing out, and even seizures and coma. Now remember, you may experience these symptoms if you're having a heart attack or stroke. Therefore, check your blood sugar if you have any of these symptoms. For more details, please refer to the section on hypoglycemia in chapter 12: Monitoring of Blood Glucose.
- Sulfonylurea failure: sulfonylurea drugs, if used alone, will require higher and higher doses of the drug over time and will eventually become ineffective in achieving good blood

glucose control. This is called sulfonylurea failure. At that point, you will be switched to insulin.

- These drugs may actually increase the risk of heart attack in diabetic patients

Starlix (generic: nateglinide), Prandin (generic: repaglinide)

Starlix (nateglinide) and Prandin (repaglinide) act by stimulating the pancreas to produce more insulin in a mechanism different from that of sulfonylurea drugs. The action of Starlix (nateglinide) and Prandin (repaglinide) lasts for four to six hours. Therefore, Starlix (nateglinide) or Prandin (repaglinide) should be taken with a meal.

Advantages

- Starlix (nateglinide) and Prandin (repaglinide) are short acting drugs taken only with meals. Therefore, the potential for low blood glucose (hypoglycemia), especially at night, is low. If you don't eat for some reason, you don't take Prandin (repaglinide) or Starlix (nateglinide). This way, you won't risk having hypoglycemia. In comparison, if a patient is on a sulfonylurea drug (which has a long duration of action), skipping a meal can lead to an episode of hypoglycemia.
- Prandin (repaglinide) is useful in patients who have kidney failure, because it is not excreted through the kidneys and, therefore, does not accumulate in the body in patients with kidney failure

Disadvantages

- These drugs do not treat insulin resistance, the underlying disease process of diabetics

- Prandin (repaglinide) and Starlix (nateglinide) are usually taken three times a day. Some patients may forget to take them properly.
- Although rare, Prandin (repaglinide) and Starlix (nateglinide) can cause low blood glucose (hypoglycemia)

Precose (generic: acarbose), Glyset (generic: miglitol)

Precose (acarbose) and Glyset (miglitol) act by decreasing glucose absorption from the intestine after eating a meal. These drugs are particularly useful if you tend to have high blood glucose levels after your meals.

Precose (acarbose) and Glyset (miglitol) can be combined with any of the other antidiabetic drugs mentioned above.

Advantages

- Precose (acarbose) and Glyset (miglitol), by themselves, do not cause low blood glucose levels (hypoglycemia)
- Precose (acarbose) and Glyset (miglitol) can help to control postmeal rises in blood glucose levels

Disadvantages

- They do not treat insulin resistance, the underlying disease process of diabetics
- If used alone, Precose (acarbose) as well as Glyset (miglitol) are weak drugs to control blood glucose levels
- Patients frequently experience gastrointestinal side effects, such as flatulence, diarrhea, and abdominal pain; even liver toxicity can develop, especially with larger doses

Caution

Liver function tests should be done every two to three months if you are on Precose (acarbose) or Glyset (miglitol).

Byetta (generic: exenatide)

Byetta (exenatide) is a newer drug in the treatment of Type 2 diabetes. Byetta (exenatide) acts by mimicking a chemical in our body known as GLP-1 (glucagon-like peptide-1). GLP-1 is one of the normally occurring hormones (chemicals) in our body, known collectively as incretins. Byetta (exenatide) has several actions that include:

- Insulin production from the pancreas in response to a glucose load from food
- Decrease in glucose output from the liver
- Slow stomach emptying. Consequently, food moves slowly from the stomach to the intestines, where absorption of food into the blood takes place. Thus, there is a slow rise in blood glucose after a meal.
- Decreased appetite

Advantages
- Byetta (exenatide) is particularly helpful to control the sharp rise in glucose after meals
- Byetta (exenatide), by itself, does not cause hypoglycemia (low blood sugar)
- Byetta (exenatide) can help you lose weight

Disadvantages

- Byetta (exenatide) does not treat insulin resistance, the underlying disease process in diabetics
- Byetta (exenatide) has to be taken by injection, like insulin
- Nausea and vomiting is a common side effect

Caution

Because Byetta (exenatide) slows stomach emptying, it may reduce the absorption of other orally administered drugs. Therefore, drugs such as antibiotics and contraceptives should be taken at least an hour before a Byetta (exenatide) injection.

Januvia (generic: sitagliptin)

Januvia (sitagliptin) is the newest drug in the treatment of Type 2 diabetes. Januvia (sitagliptin) acts by increasing the concentrations of two normally occurring chemicals in our body called incretins. These are GLP-1 (glucagon-like peptide-1) and GIP (glucose-dependent insulinotropic polypeptide). Januvia (sitagliptin) acts by:

- Producing insulin from the pancreas in response to a glucose load from food
- Decreasing glucose output from the liver

Advantages

- Januvia (sitagliptin) is particularly helpful to control the sharp rise in glucose after meals
- Januvia (sitagliptin), by itself, does not cause hypoglycemia (low blood sugar)

Disadvantages

- Januvia (sitagliptin) does not treat insulin resistance, the underlying disease process of diabetics
- Common side effects include upper respiratory tract infections (common colds) and headaches

Caution

- Januvia (sitagliptin) can cause an increase in the blood level of digoxin. Therefore, if you take digoxin, make sure to have your blood level of digoxin checked on a regular basis. Your dose of digoxin will be adjusted accordingly by your physician.
- The dose of Januvia (sitagliptin) needs to be decreased in patients with chronic kidney failure of moderate and severe degree

My Unique Approach to Antidiabetic Drugs

As itemized above, different antidiabetic drugs act through different mechanisms. Unfortunately, the underlying principle of the popular, conventional approach to the treatment of diabetes followed by most physicians is as follows: "All antidiabetic drugs are the same; start with the cheapest ones. Add another drug when one fails and move toward the more expensive ones gradually. Any drug that will control blood glucose is good enough."

I don't subscribe to that mind-set (about costs), and I don't subscribe to that approach (step-up). In contrast, I have developed my own unique approach. When I see a diabetic patient, I assess his or her severity of insulin resistance and the capacity of his or her pancreas to produce insulin. Based on the results of this assessment, I categorize an individual's diabetes as mild, moderate, or severe.

Mild Case = Hemoglobin A1c < 6.5%

Moderate Case = Hemoglobin A1c 6.5% to 8.0%

Severe Case = Hemoglobin A1c > 8.0%

Once the severity of a person's case has been established, I customize an individual treatment plan for that individual. I choose the appropriate antidiabetic drugs, regardless of their price, to achieve my goal of treating insulin resistance and not just blood glucose. Within each general category, there are, of course, all kinds of variations. You'll want to talk with your doctor about your individual case.

But before I explain how I use different antidiabetic drugs in my patients, let me re-emphasize that I not only treat diabetes but also pay close attention to other components of Insulin Resistance Syndrome, particularly cholesterol disorder and hypertension. Let me first briefly explain how I treat cholesterol disorder and hypertension in my diabetic patients. As you recall from chapter 3, patients with Type 2 diabetes often also have high blood pressure, elevated triglycerides, low HDL (good) cholesterol, and LDL (bad) cholesterol Type B, which is more harmful. Using my new treatment approach for Type 2 diabetes, not only does diabetes get under control, but HDL (good) cholesterol improves, triglycerides come down, and LDL (bad) cholesterol changes from Type B (more harmful) to Type A (less harmful). In addition, I also aim to lower LDL cholesterol to below 100 mg/dl by using a statin drug. These drugs include Zocor (simvastatin), Lipitor (atorvastatin), Crestor (rosuvastatin), Pravachol (pravastatin), Lescol (fluvastatin), and Mevacor (lovastatin). In some patients, I also use another, relatively new drug, Zetia (ezetimibe). It is also available as Vytorin as a combination of ezetimibe and simvastatin.

I treat hypertension primarily with ACE inhibitors (angiotensin converting enzyme–inhibitors) and/or ARB (angiotensin receptor blocker) drugs. These two classes of blood pressure medicines decrease insulin resistance in addition to lowering blood pressure. In comparison, beta-blockers and thiazide diuretics, which are often used to treat high blood pressure, may worsen insulin resistance. Commonly prescribed ACE-inhibitors include Altace (ramipril), Accupril (quinapril), Lotensin (benazepril), Monopril (fosinopril), Zestril or Prinivil (lisinopril), Vasotec (enalapril), Aceon (perindopril), and Capoten (captopril). Commonly prescribed ARB drugs include Diovan (valsartan), Cozaar (losartan), Avapro (irbesartan), Benicar (olmesartan), Atacand (candesartan), and Micardis (telmisartan).

Mild Cases of Type 2 Diabetes

In mild cases of Type 2 diabetes, insulin resistance is the major problem. In response to insulin resistance, the pancreas produces large quantities of insulin. This is particularly true if you have abdominal obesity. If there is any doubt about insulin production, as may happen if you are not obese, then insulin production can be assessed by checking your C-peptide (or insulin) level with a blood test. Insulin resistance takes place at three levels: fat, muscle, and liver. TZD drugs such as Actos (pioglitazone) or Avandia (rosiglitazone) treat insulin resistance at the level of fat and muscle and also have mild effects at the level of the liver. Metformin primarily treats insulin resistance at the level of the liver.

Therefore, in these early, mild diabetic patients, I target their insulin resistance by diet, exercise, vitamins, stress reduction, and the use of a TZD (thiazolidinedione) drug such as Actos (pioglitazone) or Avandia (rosiglitazone) alone. In some cases, I may add Glucophage (metformin) to the TZD drug.

Here's a case in point: Zara, a fifty-four-year-old Pakistani American woman with a history of elevated triglycerides and elevated blood glucose levels, came to see me for her fatigue. Her mother and two brothers all had Type 2 diabetes.

I gave her a two-hour oral glucose tolerance test (OGTT) with the following results:

	Baseline	One Hour	Two Hours
Blood Glucose	111 mg/dl	279 mg/dl	247 mg/dl

This test confirmed that she indeed was diabetic. She was not obese. Therefore, I checked her C-peptide level, which was high, indicating she was producing large amounts of insulin in response to insulin resistance.

I placed her on my diet combined with exercise, vitamins, stress management, and the drug Actos. Zara's diabetes is under excellent control as evidenced by her hemoglobin A1c level which has stayed under 6% over the past five years. Hemoglobin A1c is a blood test that shows your overall glucose control in the preceding three months. Zara has not developed any complications of diabetes.

Moderate Cases of Type 2 Diabetes

When Type 2 diabetes is not diagnosed for a period of time, it progresses to a more advanced stage. It is evidenced by a higher hemoglobin A1c level than individuals in mild cases. These patients often have developed some complications of diabetes by the time their diabetes is diagnosed.

As in mild cases, insulin resistance is the major problem in moderate cases of Type 2 diabetes. There is still enough insulin production by the pancreas. Therefore, I focus on treating insulin resistance in these individuals. To this end, I use my five pillar approach—diet, exercise, vitamins, stress management, and medications.

In most individuals, I chose a TZD drug such as Actos (pioglitazone) or Avandia (rosiglitazone) and a metformin, which is available as a generic as well as under various brand names such as Glucophage, Fortamet, Glumetza, or Riomet. In my clinical experience, I have found that the combination of Actos (pioglitazone) or Avandia (rosiglitazone) and a metformin is an effective way to treat insulin resistance and diabetes in a majority of moderate cases of diabetes.

o   o   o

The case of Carla, a fifty-two-year-old Caucasian female, is illustrative of all this. Carla was referred to me by her neurologist for newly diagnosed diabetes. She started experiencing tingling and numbness in her feet several years earlier. Her internist, whom she saw on a regular basis, sent her to a cardiologist for a cardiac workup for those symptoms. Her cardiologist then referred her to a podiatrist, who suspected peripheral neuropathy and sent her to a neurologist. The neurologist confirmed her peripheral neuropathy and ordered an oral glucose tolerance test to evaluate her for diabetes as the cause for peripheral neuropathy.

The results of her oral glucose tolerance test:

	Fasting	One Hour	Two Hours
Blood Glucose	133 mg/dl	266 mg/dl	207 mg/dl

These results confirmed Carla to be diabetic. Diabetes was the cause of her peripheral neuropathy. Not surprisingly, she had a family history of diabetes in one of her grandmothers, high blood pressure in her mother, and coronary heart disease in her father.

Medications

Allegra and Advair inhaler for allergies
Protonix for gastroesophageal reflux disease
Midrin for headaches

Physical Examination

Blood Pressure = 140/90 mm Hg
Weight = 256 lbs (about 100 lbs overweight)
Height = 5'6"

Laboratory Results

Fasting blood glucose = 133 mg/dl (should be 70–100 mg/dl)
HbA1c = 7.0% (should be less than 6.0%)
Triglycerides = 216 mg/dl (should be less than 150 mg/dl)
HDL Cholesterol = 44 mg/dl (should be more than 50 mg/dl in females)
LDL Cholesterol = 167 mg/dl (should be less than 100 mg/dl in diabetics)

Diagnosis

I diagnosed Carla with Insulin Resistance Syndrome, consisting of Type 2 diabetes, obesity, elevated triglyceride level, low HDL cholesterol, and high blood pressure. Her peripheral neuropathy, which had been going on for years, was most likely due to ongoing prediabetes, which had now progressed to diabetes.

Treatment

1. Diabetes

I gave Carla my recommendations on diet and exercise and discussed strategies for stress management. I placed her on Glupride Multi, a special multivitamin containing a high dose of alpha-lipoic acid, chromium picolinate, cinnamon, and coenzyme Q10. In addition, I placed her on Actos 15 mg/day and Glucophage 500 mg/day, which was gradually increased to 1000 mg twice a day.

DIABETES CONTROL

	Baseline	2 Months	11 Months	24 Months	36 Months	45 Months
Fasting Blood Glucose	133 mg/dl	107 mg/dl	105 mg/dl	118 mg/dl	99 mg/dl	103mg/dl
Hemoglobin A1c	7.0%	5.7%	5.5%	5.6%	5.9%	5.8%

2. Cholesterol

With the treatment of insulin resistance listed above, Carla's triglycerides came down and her HDL cholesterol improved remarkably. In addition to Actos and Glucophage, I placed her on Zocor 20 mg/day, primarily to lower her LDL cholesterol.

CHOLESTEROL CONTROL

	Baseline	6 Months	14 Months	26 Months	37 Months	41 Months
HDL Cholesterol	44 mg/dl	56 mg/dl	67 mg/dl	65 mg/dl	65 mg/dl	71 mg/dl
Triglycerides	216 mg/dl	94 mg/dl	76 mg/dl	103 mg/dl	77 mg/dl	67 mg/dl
LDL Cholesterol	167 mg/dl	95 mg/dl	105 mg/dl	105 mg/dl	102 mg/dl	101 mg/dl

3. Hypertension

I placed Carla on Benicar 20 mg twice a day, which has controlled her blood pressure nicely over these last four years. Her blood pressure readings remain in the range of 100–120/70–80 mm Hg.

4. Peripheral Neuropathy

During the past four years that Carla has been under my treatment, her peripheral neuropathy has not only been stable but has actually improved as evidenced by a repeat special peripheral nerve test. This result is quite amazing and exciting for me as well as her neurologist, because the usual course of diabetic peripheral neuropathy is downhill with the passage of time.

Severe Cases of Diabetes and Using My Treatment Triangle

When Type 2 diabetes is not diagnosed for an even longer period of time, it progresses to a more advanced stage as evidenced by markedly elevated hemoglobin A1c of more than 8%.

In severe cases of diabetes, in addition to insulin resistance, there is a relative decrease in insulin production by the pancreas. This decrease in insulin production is due to two reasons:

1. The toxic effect of high blood glucose on the pancreas itself. This phenomenon is called glucose toxicity. It is reversible with good control of blood glucose levels.
2. The consequence of insulin resistance on the pancreas. Patients with insulin resistance have a high level of free fatty acids, which are toxic to the pancreas. This phenomenon is known as

lipotoxicity. Free fatty acids are usually measured in research laboratories and not in a typical clinical setting. In clinical practice, we use the serum triglyceride level as an assessment of the amount of free fatty acids. If your triglyceride level is more than 150 mg/dl, you have a high level of free fatty acids.

In summary, there are three fundamental defects in severe cases of Type 2 diabetic patients:

- Insulin resistance in the muscle and fat cells
- Insulin resistance in the liver
- Decrease in the production of insulin by the pancreas relative to the insulin resistance. As a general rule, the longer the duration of diabetes, the lesser is the insulin production.

All three of these defects must be addressed to treat diabetes effectively. Picture a triangular enclosure for the angry beast we call diabetes. You can't keep it under control if you secure only one or two sides of the triangle. It will continue to go on a rampage wherever it finds an opening. You have to control all three sides of this triangle to keep it contained. I call it the treatment triangle for diabetes.

In patients with severe diabetes, I use a combination of:

- Actos (pioglitazone) or Avandia (rosiglitazone) to treat insulin resistance at the level of fat and muscle
- Metformin to reduce insulin resistance at the level of the liver
- Starlix or Prandin or a sulfonylurea drug such as glipizide or glyburide to increase insulin production
- Recently, I have started using Januvia or Byetta. These drugs increase insulin production after meals. In addition, they also slow down the rate of glucose entry from the intestines into the blood.

This is how I cover all three sides of the treatment triangle to tame the beast of diabetes in these patients. With severe diabetes, I start out with three to four drugs and gradually step down to two drugs within 6–12 months.

After about six months, I am able to either stop or substantially reduce the dose of the Starlix, Prandin, or sulfonylurea drug. By then, Actos or Avandia is having its maximum effect in lowering insulin resistance. Pancreatic function to produce insulin has also significantly improved by this time due to the decrease of glucose toxicity and lipotoxicity.

In clinical studies, TZD drugs have been shown to rejuvenate beta cells in the pancreas.[3] I see this pancreas-salvaging effect of TZD drugs (Actos, Avandia) in my diabetic patients.

By the end of a year, most of my patients are on Actos or Avandia and metformin and they continue to have good control of their diabetes.

By using this treatment triangle approach, I achieve excellent, long-lasting control in a majority of severe cases of diabetes. Also, I must emphasize that my approach to diet, exercise, vitamins, and stress management helps my patients tremendously in treating insulin resistance and controlling their diabetes. Drugs alone would not achieve these kinds of results. Remember, you have to address the five causes of insulin resistance with the corresponding five pillars of treatment in order to achieve these positive results.

o   o   o

Alfredo, a forty-two-year-old Hispanic-Japanese American, is a good example of severe diabetes that we controlled using my treatment approach. Alfredo consulted me for his newly diagnosed diabetes. Over the past year, he had experienced excessive thirst, frequent urination, and blurry vision, but he did not seek medical advice. Finally, he went to a local hospital where they found his nonfasting blood glucose to be markedly elevated at 465 mg/dl. He was sent home on Glucophage.

Alfredo's father, mother, and two grandparents all had Type 2 diabetes. His maternal grandfather had high blood pressure, coronary heart disease, and a stroke.

Physical Examination

Blood Pressure = 105/70 mm Hg
Weight = 152 lbs
Height = 5'7"
No obesity. His weight was appropriate for his height.

Laboratory Results

Fasting blood glucose = 228 mg/dl (should be 70–100 mg/dl)
HbA1c = 12.2% (should be less than 6.0%)
Triglycerides = 155 mg/dl (should be less than 150 mg/dl)
HDL Cholesterol = 37 mg/dl (should be more than 40 mg/dl in males)
LDL Cholesterol = 183 mg/dl Type B (should be less than 100 mg/dl and Type A pattern in diabetics)
ALT = 66 u/l (should be less than 45 u/l) (ALT, short for alanine aminotransferase, is a blood test for liver function. An elevated ALT means that your liver function is abnormal.)

Diagnosis

In view of his elevated triglycerides, low HDL cholesterol, Type B LDL cholesterol, and his family history, I suspected that Alfredo's diabetes was Type 2 and that he was suffering from Insulin Resistance Syndrome. However, in view of his symptoms of excessive thirst and urination and the fact that he was not overweight, I wanted to make sure that he did not have Type 1 diabetes. So I ordered a C-peptide level, which turned out to be 2.0 ng/ml (normal range = 0.8–3.1 ng/ml) indicating that indeed he had Type 2 diabetes.

His elevated ALT indicated liver inflammation from fatty liver, a complication of insulin resistance and Type 2 diabetes.

Treatment

1. Diabetes

I educated Alfredo about diabetes and Insulin Resistance Syndrome. I placed him on my diet, and advised him to walk for about thirty minutes every day. I discussed stress management with him. I placed him on Glupride Multi.

Using my treatment triangle approach, I prescribed Actos, Glucophage, and Starlix for Alfredo. Within a week, he started feeling better. Within a month, his blood glucose was coming under good control. By five months, he achieved excellent control of his diabetes. At six months, I stepped Alfredo down off of Starlix. Now, he continues to have excellent control of his diabetes on Actos and Glucophage.

DIABETES CONTROL

	Baseline	1 Month	5 Months	10 Months	21 Months	24 Months
Fasting Blood Glucose	228 mg/dl	90 mg/dl	113 mg/dl	114 mg/dl	101 mg/dl	99 mg/dl
Hemoglobin A1c	12.2%	9.0%	5.7%	5.8%	5.4%	5.3%

2. Cholesterol Control

Once I got Alfredo's insulin resistance under control, his HDL (good) cholesterol went up and his triglycerides level came down nicely. I added Zocor to lower his LDL cholesterol. Good control of insulin resistance also shifted his LDL pattern from Type B (really harmful) to Type A (less harmful).

CHOLESTEROL CONTROL

	Baseline	10 Months	14 Months
HDL Cholesterol	37 mg/dl	53 mg/dl	57 mg/dl
Triglycerides	155 mg/dl	87 mg/dl	72 mg/dl
LDL Cholesterol	183 mg/dl Type B	50 mg/dl Type A	43 mg/dl Type A

3. Weight, Blood Pressure, and ALT

During the last two years that Alfredo has been under my care, his weight has fluctuated between 153 and 165 lbs and his blood pressure between 100/70 to 120/80 mm Hg. (Last weight = 154 lbs; last blood pressure 115/80 mm Hg.)

His ALT came down to a normal level within one month and has stayed normal in the last twenty-four months.

Out-of-control Diabetes
Despite Antidiabetic Medications

As I've discussed already, most physicians continue to adhere to the popular, conventional approach to treat diabetes. In this unfortunate step-up approach, a patient is usually started on a sulfonylurea drug alone (a cheap drug), which initially controls blood glucose by increasing insulin production but does not reduce insulin resistance. As insulin resistance continues to worsen with time, the dose of the sulfonylurea drug is increased to the maximum dosage. Even the maximum dose eventually fails to control diabetes. The pancreas, exhausted in the face of mounting insulin resistance, produces smaller and smaller amounts of insulin. Eventually the pancreas fails completely.

At that point, the physician usually switches from the sulfonylurea drug to Glucophage (metformin). It does not work either, because again, only one out of three defects is being treated. Then, they often place the patient on insulin. Again, a poor strategy because insulin does not treat insulin resistance. Your diabetes stays out of control despite large doses of insulin.

o   o   o

Mahnoosh, a forty-eight-year-old Iranian American, provides us with a good example of out-of-control diabetes brought under control using my approach. Before consulting me, Mahnoosh was diagnosed with diabetes about two years prior by her internist and was placed on Glucotrol (glipizide). Initially she responded well to Glucotrol, but then her blood glucose started to rise. (To me, this was quite expected, as Glucotrol does not treat insulin resistance, which, if left untreated, continues to worsen over time.)

Then, her internist switched her from Glucotrol to Glucophage. Switching from Glucotrol to Glucophage did not control her diabetes either, primarily because, again, only one out of three sides of the triangle were being treated. This is another common mistake made by many physicians. At that point, her physician told her to go on insulin, but she decided to seek a consultation with me.

Her home blood glucose monitoring showed that her fasting blood glucose was markedly high and usually stayed in the range of 160–200 mg/dl. She felt tired all the time and had also developed tingling in her feet.

She also was diagnosed with cholesterol disorder and had been placed on Lipitor.

In her family, one uncle and one cousin had diabetes. Her father had heart disease.

Medications

Glucophage 850 mg/day
Lipitor 10 mg/day

Physical Examination

Blood Pressure = 170/80 mm Hg
Weight = 177 lbs (about 50 lbs overweight)

Treatment

1. Diabetes

Mahnoosh and I talked about the five pillars of treatment and she started to adhere to my diet, exercise, vitamins, and stress management recommendations. Using the Treatment Triangle approach, I prescribed Actos 45 mg/day and Glucovance 5/500 (a combination of glyburide 5 mg plus metformin 500 mg) for her.

At two weeks, her fasting blood glucose was 98 mg/dl and she was feeling much better. Her fatigue and the tingling in her feet were improving. I decreased her Glucovance to one tablet twice a day from three times a day.

At one month, her blood glucose was staying below 80 mg/dl with occasional low blood sugars. I stopped Glucovance and placed her on Glucophage 850 mg twice a day.

At two months, her fasting blood glucose was 123 mg/dl. She did not have any more episodes of low blood glucose.

Mahnoosh has been under my care for about six years. She continues to have excellent control of her diabetes on Actos and Glucophage. Her most recent HbA1c was 5.8%. She has not developed any complications of diabetes in the last six years.

DIABETES CONTROL

	Baseline	2 Weeks	2 Months	26 Months	31 Months
Fasting Blood Glucose	167 mg/dl	98 mg/dl	123 mg/dl	113 mg/dl	105 mg/dl
HbA1c	8.1 %	N/A	5.5%	5.5%	5.4%

2. Cholesterol Disorder

My treatment approach not only controlled her diabetes but also increased her HDL (good) cholesterol and lowered her triglycerides. I kept her on Lipitor 10 mg/day to lower her LDL cholesterol.

CHOLESTEROL CONTROL

	Baseline	2 Months	26 Months	35 Months
Total Cholesterol	167 mg/dl	176 mg/dl	199 mg/dl	165 mg/dl
LDL Cholesterol	95 mg/dl	93 mg/dl	104 mg/dl	84 mg/dl
HDL Cholesterol	52 mg/dl	51 mg/dl	71 mg/dl	60 mg/dl
Triglycerides	153 mg/dl	160 mg/dl	118 mg/dl	103 mg/dl

3. High Blood Pressure

I placed Mahnoosh on Avalide 150/12.5 mg (combination of Avapro 150 mg plus hydrochlorthiazide 12.5 mg) a day which controlled her blood pressure nicely.

BLOOD PRESSURE CONTROL

	Baseline	2 Weeks	1 Month	2 Months	31 Months	35 Months
Blood Pressure	170/80 mm Hg	120/70 mm Hg	120/70 mm Hg	125/70 mm Hg	130/70 mm Hg	120/70 mm Hg

Switching from Metformin to a Sulfonylurea Drug Does Not Work Either!

Some physicians now start out with metformin, especially now that its cost is lower. (Metformin was previously only available in brand form as Glucophage. It is now available as generic metformin and is, therefore, much less expensive.) However, if you start out with metformin alone, you're still only covering one side of the triangle. That is why you won't achieve good control of diabetes over the long term with metformin alone.

o   o   o

Christina, a thirty-six-year-old Caucasian, decided to seek an endocrine consultation for her uncontrolled diabetes. She had developed diabetes during her first pregnancy eight years earlier. After delivery, she was appropriately tested every year for diabetes. Four years ago, she was diagnosed with diabetes. She had no family history of diabetes.

Her physician started her on Glucophage, but her diabetes remained uncontrolled. Then, her physician switched her from Glucophage to glipizide, the dose of which was gradually increased to the maximum dose. However, Christina's diabetes remained out of control. Her blood glucose at home was usually around 150 mg/dl before breakfast.

Her physician told her that she probably was a Type 1 diabetic and would have to go on insulin therapy. At that point, Christina consulted me.

Physical Examination

Blood pressure = 100/70 mm Hg
Weight = 115 lbs (ideal body weight for her height)
Rest of the examination was unremarkable

Treatment

Contrary to a common misconception, Type 2 diabetes does develop in thin, lean people. Though Christina is Caucasian, it's important to note that this is especially true among Asians.

I ordered a blood test for C-peptide in order to categorize her diabetes. The test confirmed that Christina was a Type 2 diabetic and, therefore, did not need insulin therapy.

Christina and I talked about my recommendations for the five pillar approach. In addition to my diet, exercise, vitamins, and stress management advice, I utilized my treatment triangle to choose her antidiabetic drugs. I prescribed Actos, Glucophage, and glipizide for her. Later on, I switched from glipizide to Starlix because Starlix is a short acting drug that is particularly useful in controlling a rise in blood glucose after a meal.

Within five months, she achieved excellent control of her diabetes with a hemoglobin A1c of 5.7%.

Christina has been under my care for five years and continues to have excellent control of her diabetes. She has not required insulin therapy. Also, she has not developed any complications of diabetes.

Out-of-Control Diabetes Even with Multiple Drugs

Failure of a Combination of a Sulfonylurea Drug and Metformin

Even the combination of a sulfonylurea drug and Glucophage (metformin) does not work for long, as only two out of three defects are treated.

o   o   o

Consider Richard, a sixty-five-year-old Caucasian, who came to see me for his uncontrolled Type 2 diabetes. He was diagnosed with Type 2 diabetes fifteen years ago. Initially, his physician put him on glyburide and kept increasing the dose. Not surprisingly, there came a point when even the maximum dose of glyburide didn't control his diabetes.

Then, his physician added Glucophage to glyburide, but still his diabetes remained out of control. On this regimen, his fasting blood glucose had been around 200 mg/dl. His physician told him that he needed to start insulin therapy. At that point, he came to see me.

He also had a history of high blood pressure for the past twenty-five years.

His grandmother had diabetes. His father, two brothers, and one sister all had high blood pressure.

Physical examination

Blood pressure = 170/95 mm Hg
Weight = 176 lbs, Height = 5'11" (he was at his ideal body weight)
Rest of the examination was unremarkable

Medications

Glyburide 10 mg twice a day
Glucophage 1000 mg twice a day
Prinivil 5 mg once a day

Treatment

1. Diabetes

I educated Richard about my five pillars approach. Using my treatment triangle, I added Actos 45 mg/day to the Glucophage 1000 mg twice a day and glyburide 10 mg twice a day.

Within four months, Richard started turning his diabetes around. By seven months, he achieved good control of diabetes. With the passage of time, he continued to achieve even better control of his diabetes.

Seven years later, he continues to have excellent control of his diabetes as evidenced by his latest hemoglobin A1c of 5.7%. He achieved this excellent control of his diabetes without going on insulin. He has not developed any complications of diabetes.

DIABETES CONTROL

	Baseline	4 Months	7 Months	30 Months	40 Months	48 Months	84 Months
Hemoglobin A1c	8.8%	7.9%	6.7%	6.5%	6.4%	6.3%	5.7%

2. Cholesterol Disorder

With my revolutionary approach, once I got his insulin resistance under control, his HDL (good) cholesterol went up and his triglyceride level came down nicely. I added Lipitor 10 mg/day to lower his LDL cholesterol.

CHOLESTEROL CONTROL

	Baseline	7 Months	30 Months	38 Months	48 Months	80 Months
Triglycerides	201 mg/dl	157 mg/dl	62 mg/dl	52 mg/dl	82 mg/dl	56 mg/dl
HDL Cholesterol	30 mg/dl	35 mg/dl	42 mg/dl	46 mg/dl	46 mg/dl	45 mg/dl
LDL Cholesterol	156 mg/dl	84 mg/dl	89 mg/dl	70 mg/dl	73 mg/dl	69 mg/dl

3. Blood Pressure

I switched him from Prinivil to Accupril 40 mg/day as Accupril, in my opinion, is a better ACE inhibitor. At four months, I added Atacand 32 mg/day to further lower his blood pressure. Atacand is an ARB drug (angiotensin receptor blocker). Gradually his blood pressure came under excellent control. Due to insurance issues, Accupril was subsequently changed to lisinopril 40 mg/day, which is the generic name for Prinivil.

BLOOD PRESSURE CONTROL

	Baseline	4 Months	7 Months	34 Months	41 Months	48 Months	84 Months
Blood Pressure	170/90 mm Hg	170/80 mm Hg	130/80 mm Hg	135/70 mm Hg	110/70 mm Hg	140/70 mm Hg	140/60 mm Hg

Failure of a Combination of a Metformin and TZD Drug

Some physicians even try to use a combination of metformin and a TZD, (Actos or Avandia), but even this does not achieve excellent control of diabetes because only two out of three sides of the triangle are treated.

o   o   o

Mike, a sixty-eight-year-old Caucasian, consulted me for his uncontrolled diabetes. He was diagnosed with Type 2 diabetes ten years ago. He was also diagnosed with high triglycerides thirty years ago and high blood pressure twenty years ago. Over the years, he had seen several endocrinologists and dietitians. He followed the conventional diabetic diet and took his medications, but his diabetes remained out of control.

Currently, he was on metformin 1500 mg three times a day and Actos 30 mg twice a day. His fasting blood glucose values were between 250–300 mg/dl.

He complained of fatigue, numbness of toes, and excessive thirst and urination. About a year ago, he had suffered a ministroke.

His father had diabetes and hypertension and had died of a heart attack at the age of fifty-seven. Five out of his nine siblings had diabetes. His mother had hypertension.

Physical Examination

Blood Pressure = 150/110 mm Hg
Weight = 240 lbs
Height = 6'0" (about 80 lbs overweight; abdominal obesity was present)

Laboratory Results

Fasting blood glucose = 120 mg/dl (should be 70–100 mg/dl)
HbA1c = 9.6% (should be less than 6.0%)

Triglycerides = 146 mg/dl (should be less than 150 mg/dl)

HDL Cholesterol = 30 mg/dl (should be more than 40 mg/dl in males)

LDL Cholesterol = 143 mg/dl (should be less than 100 mg/dl in diabetics)

ALT = 73 u/l (should be less than 45 u/l)

Diagnosis

I diagnosed him with Insulin Resistance Syndrome consisting of Type 2 diabetes, elevated triglycerides, low HDL cholesterol, abdominal obesity, and high blood pressure.

His elevated ALT indicated liver inflammation from fatty liver, another component of insulin resistance. He had developed several complications of diabetes including peripheral neuropathy and stroke.

Treatment

1. Diabetes

I educated him about diabetes and Insulin Resistance Syndrome. I discussed my five pillars approach with him. I placed him on my diet and advised him to walk about thirty minutes a day. I discussed my stress management strategy with him. I placed him on Glupride Multi.

He was on excessive doses of metformin and Actos. The maximum daily dose of metformin is 2550 mg whereas he was taking 4500 mg/day. The maximum dose of Actos is 45 mg/day and he was on 60 mg/day.

Using my treatment triangle approach, I put him on Actos 45 mg/day, metformin 850 mg three times a day, and Starlix 120 mg three times a day.

Within three months, he achieved excellent control of diabetes as evidenced by a hemoglobin A1c of 6.0%. By this time, his ALT also normalized indicating normalization of his liver function.

He continues to have excellent control of diabetes and his liver function has stayed normal.

DIABETES CONTROL

	Baseline	1 Month	3 Months	5 Months	7 Months
Fasting Blood Glucose	120 mg/dl	127 mg/dl	129 mg/dl	122 mg/dl	101mg/dl
Hemoglobin A1c	9.6%	8.3%	6.0%	6.1%	6.2%

2. Cholesterol Disorder

At one month, his triglycerides came down to a desirable level and his HDL was going up. I added Zetia to lower his LDL cholesterol. His LDL cholesterol came down, but his HDL cholesterol also came down and his triglycerides went back up. He has not had a recent cholesterol panel since then. He will have it done in three months and we will go from there.

CHOLESTEROL CONTROL

	Baseline	1 Month	3 Months
Triglycerides	146 mg/dl	96 mg/dl	138 mg/dl
HDL Cholesterol	30 mg/dl	35 mg/dl	31 mg/dl
LDL Cholesterol	143 mg/dl	125 mg/dl	95 mg/dl

3. Hypertension

I placed him on Avapro 150 mg/day, which controlled his blood pressure well. Later, upon the request of his insurance company, it was changed to Benicar, which is also controlling his blood pressure well.

Avapro and Benicar belong to the same class of drugs known as ARBs (angiotensin receptor blockers). All ARBs are excellent drugs to control hypertension in diabetics.

HYPERTENSION CONTROL

	Baseline	1 Month	3 Months	7 Months
Blood Pressure	150/110 mm Hg	100/70 mm Hg	100/70 mm Hg	120/80 mm Hg

Remember that antidiabetic drugs are just one of the five pillars of my approach to achieving long-term, excellent control of diabetes. Most patients continue to follow a conventional diabetic diet, do not exercise, do not use appropriate vitamins, and, like most of us, have no idea how to deal with the stress of today's hectic lifestyle. It's no surprise that they continue to struggle with their diabetes.

Coming Off Insulin!

Many Type 2 diabetic patients end up on insulin primarily because most physicians continue to follow the conventional treatment approach. As you recall, the conventional treatment strategy simply tries to control blood glucose by one drug or the other without any regard as to how the drug works. Insulin resistance, the root cause of Type 2 diabetes, is not treated. Therefore, patients not only end up on insulin but also suffer the consequences of insulin resistance in the form of heart attacks, strokes, leg amputations, dementia, and other deadly complications.

My treatment approach, on the contrary, targets insulin resistance. Therefore, most of my Type 2 diabetic patients do not end up on insulin. What is even more amazing is that I am able to stop insulin even in those unfortunate Type 2 diabetic patients who are already on insulin. Not only are these patients able to come off insulin, but their diabetes also comes under much better control. In addition, this new treatment approach enables them to prevent further complications of diabetes.

The following case from my practice illustrates how I accomplish this uphill task.

o   o   o

Remember Betsy from chapter 4? If you recall, she was a fifty-five-year-old Caucasian female who came to see me with Type 2 diabetes that had been diagnosed ten years before I met her. Initially, she was on various sulfonylurea drugs (Micronase, Diabeta, Glucotrol) for a few years. Later, she was switched to insulin therapy as sulfonylurea drugs failed to control her diabetes. At the time I saw her, she was on NPH insulin 40 units plus regular insulin 20 units, in the morning and in the evening.

In addition to diabetes, she had cholesterol disorder, obesity, and high blood pressure. During those years, she also had developed heart disease, breast cancer, and peripheral neuropathy of her feet—all complications of insulin resistance.

Medications

NPH insulin 40 units plus regular insulin 20 units, in the morning and in the evening
Aspirin, Cardizem CD 120 mg twice a day
Lopid 600 mg twice a day

Physical Examination

Blood Pressure = 110/70 mm Hg
Weight = 208 lbs

Height = 5'5" (about 70 lbs overweight)
Vibration sense decreased in both feet
Rest of the examination was unremarkable

Laboratory Results

Fasting blood glucose = 167 mg/dl (should be 70–100 mg/dl)
HbA1c = 8.6% (should be less than 6.0%)
Triglycerides = 353 mg/dl (should be less than 150 mg/dl)
HDL Cholesterol = 27 mg/dl (should be more than 50 mg/dl in
  females)
LDL Cholesterol = 187 mg/dl (should be less than 100 mg/dl in
  diabetics)

Diagnosis

Betsy suffered from Insulin Resistance Syndrome, manifesting as
diabetes, high blood pressure, high triglycerides, low HDL, and
obesity. Her LDL cholesterol was also elevated. She had developed
coronary heart disease, breast cancer, and peripheral neuropathy
as complications of insulin resistance and diabetes. A twenty-four-
hour urinary albumin excretion turned out to be markedly elevated at 776 mg (should be less than 25 mg in 24 hours), indicating she had also developed significant kidney disease due to
uncontrolled diabetes. She was on her way to kidney dialysis.

Treatment

1. Diabetes

I discussed my five pillars approach with Betsy and she began to
change her diet, exercise, and better manage her stress. She also
started taking a Glupride Multi.

Initially I continued her on insulin and added Rezulin 400 mg/day. Rezulin was the first TZD drug released in the U.S. and had just become available. Later, Rezulin was withdrawn from the U.S. market due to a number of cases of severe liver toxicity associated with its use. Betsy, however, did not have any problems with Rezulin.

I later switched her from Rezulin to Actos 45 mg/day. Actos and Avandia are currently the available TZD drugs in the U.S. They have been used since 1999 and do not cause any excessive liver toxicity.

TZD drugs take about six months to exert their maximum effects. Therefore, at six months, I stopped her regular insulin and then at nine months, I stopped her NPH insulin. At this point I added Glucotrol XL 20 mg/day.

Later, I added Glucophage 1000 mg twice a day, Prandin 2 mg three times a day, and stopped her Glucotrol XL.

Over the last ten years, she continues to have excellent control of her diabetes on Actos, Glucophage, and Prandin. Not only did she come off insulin, but she also achieved much better control of her diabetes.

DIABETES CONTROL

	Baseline	1 Year	2 Years	3 Years	4 Years	5 Years
Fasting Blood Glucose	167 mg/dl	140 mg/dl	128 mg/dl	156 mg/dl	111 mg/dl	119 mg/dl
HgA1c	8.6%	8.5%	7.2%	8.4%	8.2%	6.1%

	6 Years	7 Years	8 Years	9 Years	10 Years
Fasting Blood Glucose	106 mg/dl	113 mg/dl	133 mg/dl	117 mg/dl	118 mg/dl
HgA1c	6.6%	5.9%	6.3%	5.6%	6.2%

2. Cholesterol Disorder

My new approach not only controlled her diabetes but also increased her HDL (good) cholesterol and lowered her triglycerides.

At five months, I stopped her Lopid as Rezulin was in full action by this time.

I kept her on Zocor to control her LDL cholesterol. Later Zocor was switched to Lipitor per request of her insurance company. Both Zocor and Lipitor are excellent drugs to lower LDL cholesterol.

CHOLESTEROL CONTROL

	Baseline	5 Months	6 Months	11 Months	31 Months	66 Months	71 Months
Triglycerides	353 mg/dl	286 mg/dl	165 mg/dl	181 mg/dl	168 mg/dl	113 mg/dl	101 mg/dl
HDL Cholesterol	27 mg/dl	32 mg/dl	30 mg/dl	38 mg/dl	37 mg/dl	45 mg/dl	50 mg/dl
LDL Cholesterol	187 mg/dl	141 mg/dl	104 mg/dl	125 mg/dl	86 mg/dl	83 mg/dl	90 mg/dl

3. Kidney Disease

Betsy had developed significant diabetic kidney disease as evidenced by marked urinary albumin excretion of 776 mg in twenty-four hours (normal being less than 25 mg). Fortunately, we were able to normalize her urinary albumin excretion by employing my treatment strategy that focuses on aggressive control of insulin resistance. I also started her on Accupril 40 mg/day which is an ACE inhibitor and also helps diabetic patients with kidney disease.

KIDNEY CONTROL

	Baseline	6 Months	11 Months	31 Months
Twenty-four-hour Urinary Albumin Excretion	776 mg	432 mg	420 mg	15 mg

Her blood pressure remained under good control throughout this period.

CHAPTER 10

Treating Type 1 Diabetes

Though there are some experimental therapies being researched and tested today (see information about islet cell transplantation on page 166), insulin therapy is still the main treatment for Type 1 diabetic patients at this time.

The Rationale of Insulin Therapy

In nondiabetics, the pancreas produces insulin all the time, even in a fasting state, at a rate of about 1 unit per hour. After eating a meal, the pancreas produces additional pulses of insulin to deal with the extra load of glucose in the meal.

In Type 1 diabetics, of course, the pancreas does not produce insulin either in the fasting state or after a meal.

With insulin therapy, you can create a continuous level of insulin by administering a long-acting insulin once a day and also regulate the glucose spike that comes with each meal by administering a short-acting insulin before each meal.

Types of Insulin

Let me first explain the various types of insulin available today:

- A long-acting insulin provides a basal—or continuous base of—insulin level in the body all the time
- A short-acting insulin before each meal provides coverage for that particular meal

VARIOUS TYPES OF LONG-ACTING INSULIN

Generic Name	Brand Name	Onset of Action	Peak of Action	Duration of Action
Glargine	Lantus	3–4 hours	No peak	About 24 hours
Ultralente	Humulin U	3–4 hours	Variable peak	Up to 28 hours
NPH	Humulin N, Novolin N	2–3 hours	6–8 hours	12–16 hours, up to 24 hours
Lente	Humulin L, Novolin L	2–3 hours	6–8 hours	12–16 hours, up to 24 hours

NPH and lente are also known as intermediate-acting insulin. A newly marketed long-acting insulin is detemir with the brand name of Levemir. Its properties are similar to those of NPH insulin.

VARIOUS TYPES OF SHORT-ACTING INSULIN

Generic Name	Brand Name	Onset of Action	Duration of Action
Lispro	Humalog	30–90 minutes	3–4 hours
Aspart	Novolog	40–50 minutes	3–4 hours
Regular	Humulin R, Novolin R	1–2 hours	5–8 hours

A newly marketed short-acting insulin is glulisine with the brand name of Apridia. Its properties are similar to those of Humalog and Novolog.

For convenience, combination insulin—some short-acting, some long-acting—are also available.

MIXTURE OF INSULIN

Brand Name	Insulin Combination	Onset of Action	Duration of Action
Humalog Mix 75/25	75% lispro protamine suspension and 25% lispro	30 minutes	12 hours
Humulin 70/30	70% NPH and 30% regular	1–2 hours	12–24 hours
Humulin 50/50	50% NPH and 50% regular	1–2 hours	12–24 hours
Novolog Mix 70/30	70% aspart protamine and 30% aspart	30 minutes	12 hours

Note: the time course of action of any insulin may vary considerably in different patients or at different times in the same patient. The duration of action depends on dose, site of injection, blood supply, temperature, and physical activity.

Long-Acting Insulin

Lantus (glargine) and Humulin U (ultralente) have a slower onset and longer duration of action than Humulin N/Novolin N (NPH) or Humulin L/Novolin L (lente).

NPH, lente, ultralente, and detemir have a peak of action that is undesirable as it can cause low blood glucose unexpectedly. On the other hand, glargine doesn't have any peak of action, making it the most desirable long-acting insulin at the present time.

Glargine insulin needs to be given only once a day and provides a good basal level.

Ultralente is also given as a once-a-day injection.

NPH or lente are also known as intermediate-acting insulin
and are generally given twice a day, usually before breakfast and
at bedtime (or dinner time).

Short-Acting Insulin

Short-acting insulin, such as Humalog (lispro), Novolog (aspart),
Apridia (glulisine), or regular insulin, is used before each meal to
provide premeal boluses of insulin.

I prefer to prescribe Humalog (lispro), Novolog (aspart), or
Apridia (glulisine) over regular insulin because these newer types
of insulin have a very rapid onset of action. A patient can take
the injection of lispro, aspart, or glulisine just before eating their
meal. However, with regular insulin, you need to wait for about
thirty to sixty minutes after the insulin shot before eating your
meal. Sometimes, patients take their regular insulin shot and then
forget to eat or wait for a long time in a restaurant for their food.
This places them at a high risk for low blood sugar (also known
as hypoglycemia or insulin reaction).

Humalog (lispro), Novolog (aspart), and Apridia (glulisine)
have another advantage in that they are out of your system in
about four to five hours as compared to regular insulin, which
hangs around in the body for about eight hours. The shorter
duration of action of lispro, aspart, and glulisine reduces the
risk of low blood sugar before the next meal as compared to
regular insulin.

Regular insulin at dinner time is usually responsible for low
blood sugar in the middle of the night. All short-acting insulin
should be avoided at bedtime.

You need to inject Humalog, Novolog, Apridia, or regular insulin before each meal.

If you administer your insulin therapy via shots, it's important to know that you can draw a short-acting insulin and a long-acting/intermediate-acting insulin in the same syringe. For example, you can draw Humalog and NPH in the same syringe before breakfast. Draw Humalog first and then NPH.

However, Lantus is an exception to this mixing. *You cannot mix Lantus (glargine) and another insulin in the same syringe.*

Administering Insulin

You can give yourself insulin in one of the following ways:

- Insulin shots
- Insulin pump
- Insulin inhalation

For your specific case, you'll need to discuss the pros and cons of each option with your physician. To prepare you for a meaningful conversation with your physician, here's what you need to know about your options:

Insulin Shots

Insulin shots deliver insulin to the body via an injection under the skin. You can give yourself an insulin shot with a traditional insulin syringe or with the relatively new technology of an insulin pen. Insulin pens are becoming popular because of their convenience—the pens are prefilled with insulin so that you don't have to take the time to draw insulin from a bottle. You still need to calculate the dose of insulin to be administered each time you use a pen.

If you use insulin shots, you must administer an injection before each meal. You must also check your blood glucose level before each insulin shot in order to best assess how much insulin to administer.

Advantages

- Insulin shots are a tested delivery system: we have the longest clinical experience with this form of insulin therapy
- With the help of a nurse, a diabetes educator, or a physician, it's pretty easy to learn how to give yourself an insulin shot
- Insulin shots are relatively inexpensive compared to other forms of insulin therapy

Disadvantages

- Although new needles are extra fine and much less painful than previous ones, some people still report that insulin shots are painful
- Having to give yourself multiple shots a day can be inconvenient

If you and your physician determine that insulin shots are the best form of insulin treatment for you, your physician or a nurse will teach you how to draw insulin from a bottle and give yourself insulin shots under the skin. The best places for insulin shots are the stomach or a thigh. You can also inject in the buttocks or an arm, but generally the stomach or a thigh enables the best insulin absorption. To avoid bruising, scar tissue (which inhibits insulin absorption), and for best insulin absorption, it's important to rotate your injection site each time you give yourself an insulin shot.

Insulin Pens

Insulin pens, which come prefilled, are rapidly becoming popular. They make it easier for diabetics to administer insulin, especially in situations such as at school or in a restaurant or office. Insulin pens are an especially good choice for children because they are self-contained and less cumbersome than insulin vials and syringes.

Insulin Shot/Pen Doses

Your physician will calculate the initial dose of long-acting insulin and short-acting insulin for you.

Thereafter, you will need to be educated on how to adjust the dose of short-acting insulin according to the type of meal you are about to eat, your level of blood glucose before the meal, and your level of activity after the meal. As a general rule, 1 unit of short-acting insulin will cover 10–15 g of carbohydrates. I tell my patients to decrease the dose if a high level of exercise such as jogging is planned after the meal. I also provide my patients with a detailed sliding scale as a guide to further adjust the dose of short-acting insulin before each meal. Ask your physician about providing you with something similar.

On each office visit, your blood glucose values should be reviewed and insulin doses should be further fine-tuned by your physician.

Insulin Pumps

Via a needle inserted under the skin and attached to a beeper-shaped pump that can hook to a belt loop, an insulin pump delivers insulin under the skin continuously. You program the pump to automatically administer an individualized basal rate of insulin throughout the day and night. After checking your blood glucose, you must also manually prompt the pump to administer a bolus of insulin before each meal.

You can program more than one basal rate, depending upon your individual needs. For example, some patients need to have two basal rates: one from 9 a.m. to 3 a.m. and then another higher basal rate from 3 a.m. to 9 a.m. to provide coverage for the dawn phenomenon.

At dawn, many diabetics have an increase in blood glucose due to a surge of three hormones in the body: growth hormone, cortisol, and catecholamines. All three of these hormones cause an increase in blood glucose. This is known as the dawn phenomenon.

Only short-acting insulin is used in an insulin pump to provide both a continuous, basal rate as well as premeal boluses.

Advantages

- The biggest advantage of an insulin pump is that it provides greater flexibility in timing of meals. You don't have to eat at a particular time as is the case with insulin injection therapy. You can even skip a meal without the fear of low blood sugar because, in an insulin pump, you don't use any long-acting insulin and only a small dose of short-acting insulin is being administered at a continuous, basal rate. You give a large dose of short-acting insulin in the form of a bolus only when you eat a meal. If you skip a meal, you don't give yourself a bolus and therefore don't run the risk of low blood sugar.
- Patients who have wide swings in their blood glucose values on insulin shots generally do much better by switching to an insulin pump

- Pregnant patients also are good candidates for an insulin pump

Disadvantages

- The learning curve: an insulin pump requires a certain level of learning skills on the part of the patient. The pump is like any technical gadget—you need to learn its various prompts thoroughly. For example, you must learn how to set the basal rate/rates, how to give boluses, and how to load the insulin reservoir in the pump. You must be able to take good care of your insulin pump and its accessories.
- The pump needle must be changed every three days—you will still need to insert a needle under your skin each time
- You must be motivated and vigilant in order to avoid and recognize complications that can occur with the use of the insulin pump, such as skin infections and mechanical failures
- Insulin pumps come with an increased risk of skin infection at the needle site. If not treated promptly, an infection at the needle site can lead to a rapid rise in blood glucose levels and even a life-threatening medical emergency, such as diabetic ketoacidosis (DKA).
- Pump mechanical failure can lead to cessation of insulin delivery and your blood glucose can rise rapidly. This situation can potentially throw you into a life-threatening medical emergency, diabetic ketoacidosis (DKA). Therefore, you need to keep a supply of insulin shots on hand for emergency situations, such as when your insulin pump or its tubing is not functioning properly.
- The insulin pump is much more expensive than insulin shots
- Some patients don't like having the pump attached to them—the pump might appear lumpy under clothing, creating cosmetic problems for some patients

Getting Started on an Insulin Pump

Once you decide to use an insulin pump, your physician will arrange for a nurse to spend time with you to educate you about your insulin pump. The nurse will familiarize you with the insulin pump and its accessories.

You then start a test period. For about three or four days, you wear an insulin pump, but instead of insulin, saline (salt water) runs through the system.

Once you feel comfortable with the operation of the pump, you go back to your physician to initiate your insulin therapy.

Insulin Pump Doses

The total daily dose of insulin for an insulin pump is about seventy five percent of the total daily dose that you take in the form of injections. Fifty percent of this dose is provided as the basal rate for the twenty-four-hour period and the other fifty percent is divided into three doses, one before each meal.

In the first week, you need to check your blood glucose before each meal, as well as at bedtime and at 3 a.m. Thereafter—if you have your pump and your blood glucose levels under control—you will likely only have to check your blood glucose before each meal.

Adjusting Pump Doses

As mentioned above, there is a certain learning curve when you use an insulin pump. You can't assume that your diabetes is now on autopilot! Depending on your blood glucose values, your physician may make further adjustments to your basal rate as well as boluses before meals. For example, in my patients, if early morning blood glucose values are high, I add another higher basal rate for the hours between 3 a.m. and 9 a.m. to cover the dawn phenomenon.

I also recommend further adjustments in the dose of boluses according to a patient's blood glucose level before a meal, the amount of carbohydrates in the meal, and the level of activity planned after the meal. I tell my patients to decrease the dose of bolus if a high level of exercise such as jogging is planned after the meal.

When using an insulin pump, it's especially important to learn carbohydrate counting so that you can accurately administer a bolus before each meal. A dietitian can help you in this regard. As a general rule, 1 unit of insulin is needed to cover 10–15 g of carbohydrates. But you will need to figure out how many grams of carbohydrates get covered by 1 unit of insulin, in your case.

Insulin by Inhalation

The newest development in insulin delivery systems is insulin by inhalation. Currently there is only one brand of inhaled insulin on the market—Exubera. Exubera is a synthetic human insulin in the form of inhalation powder. It is a rapid-acting insulin (similar to Humalog or Novolog taken by subcutaneous injection). Its duration of action is similar to regular insulin by subcutaneous injection.

In clinical trials, insulin absorption through the lungs appears to be as good as through the skin.

In Type 1 diabetics, Exubera should be used only as short-acting insulin. You'll still need a long-acting insulin by subcutaneous (under the skin) injection.

Advantages

- You avoid the pain of multiple insulin shots
- You don't need to worry about the potential mechanical problems of an insulin pump

Disadvantages

- Insulin delivery through the lungs is a new delivery system. We don't know how it's going to affect lung function in the long term. In clinical trials, there was a small decrease in the lung function in patients treated with Exubera. Therefore, your physician must check your lung function before initiating Exubera, again after six months of therapy, and then annually even if there appear to be no respiratory problems.
- In short-term clinical trials, cough was a common side effect that occurs within seconds to minutes after Exubera inhalation. Other adverse events included shortness of breath, chest pain, sore throat, nose bleed, and dry mouth.
- Exubera must not be used by smokers or by former smokers who discontinued smoking cigarettes less than six months prior to starting Exubera. If you start or resume smoking while on Exubera, you must stop Exubera and administer insulin through other methods as outlined above.
- Exubera must not be used in patients with underlying lung diseases such as asthma, emphysema, or any other lung disease
- In children, the long-term safety and effectiveness of Exubera has not been established. In my opinion, it should not be used in children until we have long-term safety data.
- Hypoglycemia, like other insulin therapies, is a significant risk

New Developments in the
Treatment of Type 1 Diabetes

Symlin (generic: pramlintide)

Symlin is a relatively new treatment for Type 1 diabetics as well as a therapy for people with Type 2 diabetes that require insulin. Symlin is not insulin. It is a synthetic analogue of amylin, a hormone that is normally secreted along with insulin by the beta cells of the pancreas. Amylin decreases glucose production by the liver, decreases the rate at which food passes from the stomach to the intestines, and also reduces appetite. Through these actions, amylin prevents a sharp increase in blood glucose after a meal. In Type 1 diabetics, amylin is no longer present. Symlin has the same actions as amylin.

However, Symlin is not a replacement for insulin. It is used in addition to insulin to further control blood glucose levels after a meal.

Symlin must be taken before meals, in addition to short-acting insulin such as Humalog, Novolog, apridia, or regular insulin.

Like insulin, Symlin needs to given by injection. However, insulin and Symlin *cannot* be mixed in the same syringe. Insulin and Symlin need to be given by separate injections.

Symlin has *not* been tested in children.

Caution

Symlin, in combination with insulin, can cause severe hypoglycemia. Therefore, you should not use Symlin if:

- You frequently experience hypoglycemia
- You cannot tell when your blood sugar is low (hypoglycemia unawareness)

- You do not check your blood glucose before and after every meal and at bedtime
- You do not see your doctor at least every two months

Side Effects

Symlin often causes nausea. If you already suffer from slow stomach emptying (a diabetic complication known as gastroparesis), you should not be on Symlin. Other side effects include vomiting, headache, weakness, dizziness, and allergic reaction.

At this time, we have very limited experience with Symlin at the Jamila Diabetes & Endocrine Medical Center. Therefore, I can't give you my complete opinion about this new drug.

Insulin Resistance Syndrome in Type 1 Diabetics

Some Type 1 diabetics slowly develop Insulin Resistance Syndrome as they get older, gain weight, and adopt a sedentary lifestyle. A typical young, thin, Type 1 diabetic patient requires about 30 to 40 units of insulin per twenty-four hours. If you use more than 40 units of insulin per each twenty-four-hour period, you probably have insulin resistance. Insulin resistance places you at high risk for cardiovascular events such as heart attacks and strokes.

My unique approach to treating Insulin Resistance Syndrome is discussed in chapters 5–9. This approach consists of five pillars: diet, exercise, stress management, vitamins, and medications. The medications I use include a TZD (thiazolidinedione) drug such as Actos (pioglitazone) or Avandia (rosiglitazone). These drugs treat insulin resistance. For more information about Actos and Avandia, please refer to page 108. For more information about Insulin Resistance Syndrome, please refer to chapter 2.

o   o   o

Peter, a Caucasian male, was diagnosed with diabetes at the age of six. For a number of years, he had been on an insulin pump and under the care of another endocrinologist. At the young age of forty-four, Peter was admitted to the hospital with a heart attack.

When I met him in the hospital, Peter's hemoglobin A1c was 7.1%, indicating that his diabetes had been uncontrolled for some time. His premeal blood glucose levels were usually 90–140 mg/dl and his two-hour postmeal blood glucose values were 200–250 mg/dl.

Peter's brother also had Type 1 diabetes. His father died of a heart attack at the age of forty-three. His mother died of a stroke at the age of seventy-five. Peter had recently started taking Lipitor for his cholesterol disorder.

Medications

Regular insulin via insulin pump
Lipitor 10 mg/day
Lopressor 25 mg twice a day (a beta-blocker)
Plavix 75 mg/day (a blood thinner)
Aspirin (a blood thinner)
Accupril 10 mg/day
Ibuprofen 800 mg as needed for chronic back pain

Physical Examination

Blood pressure = 110/60 mm Hg
Weight = 172 lbs
Height = 5'7" (about 10 lbs overweight)

Laboratory Results

Fasting Blood Glucose = 95 mg/dl (should be 70–100 mg/dl)

Hemoglobin A1c = 7.1% (should be less than 6.0%)

HDL cholesterol = 51 mg/dl (should be more than 40 mg/dl in males)

Triglycerides = 102 mg/dl (should be less than 150 mg/dl)

LDL cholesterol = 119 mg/dl (should be less than 100 mg/dl in diabetics)

Management

Peter's basal rate for regular insulin was 2.3 units/hour between 8:00 a.m. and midnight and then 0.8 units/hour between midnight and 8:00 a.m. He gave himself boluses before each meal according to carbohydrate counting.

What struck me was that Peter was on too much insulin for a Type 1 diabetic. His basal rate gave him a total of 43 units of regular insulin in a twenty-four-hour period. In addition, he gave boluses of about 10–15 units before each meal, adding another 30 to 45 units of regular insulin for every twenty-four-hour period. His total insulin intake over a twenty-four-hour period was about 70 to 90 units. He had developed insulin resistance, which brought on coronary artery disease and a heart attack at a relatively young age.

In view of his strong family history of cardiovascular disease, I checked Peter for some cardiac risk factors—Lp(a) and homocysteine levels—tests that had not been done on him before. Peter's Lp(a) turned out to be elevated at 49 mg/dl (normal being less than 10 mg/dl). His homocysteine level was 8.0 Umol/L (normal being less than 12 Umol/L).

Lp(a) is a strong risk factor for cardiovascular disease. It is genetic in nature and indicates ongoing insulin resistance. It is difficult to treat. Niacin is one option, which in diabetics is not a good option, as it can further increases blood glucose by increasing insulin resistance. Also, it often causes flushing of the face, which is quite bothersome for many patients. Niacin may also cause liver damage in some patients. Actos (pioglitazone), a drug that treats insulin resistance, decreases Lp(a) and also has beneficial effects on coronary artery disease. So, I decided to place Peter on Actos.

Peter was very well educated about his insulin pump. I changed his regular insulin to Humalog for his pump and advised him to change his basal rate according to his blood glucose levels.

A month later, Peter's basal insulin rate from 8 a.m. to midnight was down to 1.4 units/hour, while his basal rate from midnight to 8 a.m. was still 0.8 unit/hour. His total twenty-four-hour basal insulin dose came down from 43 units to 28 units.

Complications of Treatment for Type 1 Diabetes

Despite the development of a variety of insulin, treatment of Type 1 diabetics in real life is often challenging for the patient as well as physician. The biggest problem is hypoglycemia. Severe hypoglycemia with seizures and loss of consciousness is a terrifying experience for patients as well as their family members. Once you have experienced an episode of severe hypoglycemia, you don't want it to ever happen again. As a result, you keep your blood glucose relatively high. Unfortunately, these uncontrolled blood glucose levels, in the long run, can cause complications of diabetes.

Treatments on the Horizon

Islet Cell Transplantation

An experimental procedure known as islet cell transplantation holds the potential for a cure for Type 1 diabetes. In islet cell transplantation, insulin-producing beta cells are taken from a donor's pancreas and transferred into a person with diabetes. Once transplanted, the donor islets should begin to make and release insulin, actively regulating the level of glucose in the diabetic's blood.

For many years, islet cell transplantation has been the focus of scientific research. The problem for researchers is how to prevent the rejection of the transplanted beta cells by the body's immune system. In the last decade, there has been some progress in this area. A few years ago, researchers in Canada came up with a special protocol, known as the Edmonton protocol, to prevent this rejection of the beta cells. Now several medical centers in the U.S. are testing this Edmonton protocol.

Stem cell research also looks promising as a possible cure for Type 1 diabetes some day.

Please refer to chapter 12 for Monitoring of Blood Glucose in Type 1 Diabetics.

PART THREE

PREVENTING, STOPPING, AND EVEN REVERSING COMPLICATIONS OF DIABETES

CHAPTER 11

Managing Complications of Diabetes

Though my five pillar treatment approach should bring your diabetes under good control, it's important to understand the possible complications that can arise from your disease (or that may have already arisen) and to understand the further treatment tools available to you to prevent, stop, or even reverse these complications. This chapter outlines the common complications that arise from diabetes—both Type 1 and Type 2—and should provide you a good base of information from which to begin or continue a conversation with your physician about managing your disease.

Diabetes is a disease of complications, affecting almost every part of your body. As a diabetic, you're at a high risk for a number of complications, regardless of whether you require insulin or not. Don't be lulled into thinking that Type 2 diabetes—what many consider the "good kind" because you are not on insulin shots—leaves you at any less risk for complications. A major part of taking charge of your diabetes is to understand your risks and insist that your treatment manages them.

The list of frequent diabetes complications includes heart disease, stroke, blindness, amputation, kidney failure, peripheral neuropathy, impotence, and fatty liver, a condition that may lead to cirrhosis. These deadly complications develop insidiously over a long period of time. That is why patients often don't fully comprehend the devastating effects of diabetes until it's too late.

The good news—as I've stated earlier—is that my treatment approach can help prevent these horrendous complications. You can also stop and even reverse the downhill course of some of these complications after they have developed. Again, the key is to understand how these complications develop and how your treatment for diabetes should include measures to stave off these complications. What follows here is information about each of the major complications of diabetes.

A Message for Smokers

Diabetics who smoke have a markedly increased risk for developing complications of diabetes. So next time you light up, remember that the smoke is fueling the fire of complications. Read this chapter and then take a moment to meditate about the path you are on. Maybe if you truly comprehend what lies ahead on this road, you can find the strength to commit to quitting smoking.

Heart Disease in Diabetics

Coronary heart disease develops due to narrowing of the blood vessels, a process known as atherosclerosis. Atherosclerosis develops slowly over a number of years. Then one day, a clot forms at the site of the narrowed blood vessel and acutely shuts down the blood flow to a portion of the heart. This is what causes an acute heart attack or, technically speaking, angina (a minor episode without any damage to the heart muscle) or acute myocardial infarction (a prolonged episode with damage to the heart muscle).

The root cause for coronary heart disease in a majority of diabetics is Insulin Resistance Syndrome (IRS). Heart disease and heart attacks are preventable, but only with proper evaluation and treatment of IRS. If you have the risk factors for IRS—abdominal obesity, high blood pressure, low HDL cholesterol, high triglycerides, Type B LDL cholesterol, or elevated CRP (C-reactive protein), you and your physician need to target IRS and treat it.

How Insulin Resistance Puts You at a High Risk for Heart Attack

1. The Effects of High Levels of Insulin

A person with Insulin Resistance Syndrome has a higher than normal level of insulin in the bloodstream, which in turn stimulates growth of smooth muscle cells in the walls of the coronary arteries. This causes thickening and stiffness of the arterial walls, which contributes to narrowing of the coronary blood vessels: atherosclerosis.

2. High Blood Pressure

High blood pressure, a component of IRS, is present in most diabetics and is known to cause narrowing of the arterial blood vessels, including arteries of the heart. Blood pressure higher than 115/80 mm Hg increases your risk for a heart attack. Blood pressure above 130/85 mm Hg is called hypertension. A healthy blood pressure is less than 115/80 mm Hg in most individuals.

High insulin levels, due to insulin resistance, causes high blood pressure by the following mechanisms:

- It causes thickening of arterial walls, which then become stiff
- Increased resistance to blood flow through the stiff blood vessels leads to an increase in blood pressure
- It causes retention of sodium and water from the kidneys, which then leads to high blood pressure
- It stimulates the sympathetic nervous system, which causes constriction of blood vessels, which then leads to high blood pressure

3. High Triglycerides and Low HDL Cholesterol

A high level of triglycerides and a low level of HDL (good) cholesterol, both of which are components of IRS, are present in most diabetics.

In healthy individuals, one of the functions of insulin is to suppress the breakdown of fat from the fat cells into the blood stream. This action of insulin is hampered in individuals with insulin resistance. As a result there is an exaggerated breakdown of fat from the fat cells. The product of this fat breakdown is called free fatty acids. Thus, in diabetics with insulin resistance, there is a high level of free fatty acids in the blood. The liver takes up these free fatty acids and converts them into VLDL cholesterol (very low density lipoproteins). These cholesterol particles are rich in triglycerides, which is why individuals with insulin resistance have a high level of triglycerides.

When VLDL particles interact with HDL particles, VLDL exchanges its triglycerides for the cholesterol of HDL particles. This results in a decrease in HDL cholesterol. These triglycerides-enriched HDL particles also break down easily, which further lowers HDL level. That is why diabetics with insulin resistance end up with low HDL cholesterol.

HDL cholesterol works as a scavenger by cleaning out the cholesterol deposited in the walls of blood vessels. That is why HDL cholesterol is known as the "good" cholesterol. If your HDL is low, there will be less cleansing of the cholesterol buildup in the vessel wall. Therefore, a low level of HDL cholesterol is a major risk factor for narrowing of coronary blood vessels.

VLDL particles also give rise to the formation of another cholesterol particle known as IDL (intermediate density lipoprotein), which then converts to LDL (low density lipoproteins). VLDL, IDL, and LDL particles deposit in the arterial wall, which causes narrowing of the vessel wall.

4. An Increase in Type B LDL Cholesterol Particles

LDL (bad) cholesterol consists of two subpopulations:

- Large, fluffy particles (Type A)
- Small, dense particles (Type B)

Type B particles deposit more easily inside the blood vessel wall than Type A particles and, therefore, are more harmful.

In diabetic patients with insulin resistance, there is a predominance of the more harmful Type B particles, which again leads to narrowing of the coronary blood vessels.

5. An Increased Tendency for Clot Formation and Decreased Ability to Break Clots

In diabetics with insulin resistance, there is a high level of several clotting factors, including fibrinogen levels in the blood, which increases the risk for blood clot formation.

In addition, these patients also have a decreased ability to break up blood clots. This happens due to a high level of a substance known as PAI–1, short for plasminogen activator inhibitor-1.

Consequently, diabetics are at a high risk for blood clot formation and have a decreased ability to break up these clots. When a clot forms in an already narrowed coronary blood vessel, a person might suffer an acute heart attack.

6. An Elevated Highly Sensitive CRP (C-reactive protein) Level

A high level of C-reactive protein indicates ongoing inflammation in the blood vessel wall. Inflammatory cells are present in the atherosclerotic plaque inside the blood vessel wall. When inflamed, these plaques can easily rupture. A ruptured plaque attracts clotting factors. A blood clot forms at the site of a ruptured plaque, which then causes an acute shutdown of blood flow that may result in an acute heart attack. A high level of CRP, therefore, indicates a significantly higher risk for a heart attack. Diabetics with insulin resistance usually have a high level of CRP.

7. Endothelial Dysfunction

The endothelium, the lining of the blood vessel wall, produces a number of substances, a balance of which is important for its healthy functioning. A number of these substances can cause constriction of the vessel wall (vasoconstriction), while others cause a dilatation of the vessel wall (vasodilatation). In healthy individuals, there is a fine balance between these two processes.

Diabetics with insulin resistance have a disruption in this balance in such a way that there is more vasoconstriction and less vasodilatation. This endothelial dysfunction causes further narrowing of the blood vessels.

Heart Attacks Happen Even After Angioplasty

As all of the above indicates, narrowing of coronary blood vessels is a complex process. It develops over a period of years due to underlying Insulin Resistance Syndrome.

To recap, the process of narrowing of the coronary arteries consists of:

• Deposition of cholesterol in the wall of the coronary arteries
• Proliferation of a variety of cells in the wall of the coronary arteries
• Damage to the lining of the coronary arteries (endothelial dysfunction)

Angioplasty, as well as stent placement, temporarily opens up the narrowed blood vessel but has no effect on the cholesterol buildup inside the wall of the blood vessel.

After an angioplasty, if appropriate drug therapy is not instituted to treat the disease process inside the wall of the blood vessel, it will shut down again. About half of all patients who receive angioplasties experience a recurrence of blockage within six months. An angioplasty is a temporary fix. It must be followed by aggressive drug treatment of the underlying disease process.

o   o   o

Remember George from the introduction? When I met George, he was sixty-nine years old and had already undergone three angioplasties within two years. His father and uncle had diabetes, and over the prior twenty years, he himself had been diagnosed with diabetes, high blood pressure, cholesterol disorder, and congestive heart failure.

His physician treated his diabetes in the usual conventional way: initially he was on glyburide. When even the maximum doses of glyburide failed to control his blood glucose, George was switched to insulin injections.

Medications

Insulin 70/30, 40 units in the morning and 35 units in the evening
Procardia XL 60 mg/day, Vasotec 15 mg twice a day, Zocor 20 mg/day
Aspirin 325 mg once a day, digoxin 0.25 mg once a day
Lasix 40 mg twice a day, K-Dur 20 meq twice a day
Ticlid 250 mg twice a day(a blood thinner)

Physical Examination

Blood Pressure = 148/70 mm Hg
Weight = 253 lbs
He was 50 lbs overweight; abdominal obesity was present

Laboratory Results

Fasting blood glucose = 169 mg/dl (should be less than 100 mg/dl)
Hemoglobin A1c = 11.2% (should be less than 6.0%) (Hemoglobin A1c measures overall control of blood glucose in the last three months)
Triglycerides = 962 mg/dl (should be less than 150 mg/dl)
HDL cholesterol = 22 mg/dl (should be more than 40 mg/dl in males)
LDL cholesterol = Could not be calculated due to high triglyceride level

Diagnosis

I diagnosed George with Insulin Resistance Syndrome as evidenced by Type 2 diabetes, low HDL cholesterol, high triglycerides, obesity, and high blood pressure. He had clearly developed coronary artery disease as a complication of this syndrome. His diabetes was severely uncontrolled despite being on insulin therapy.

Treatment

My treatment plan targeted all the components of his IRS—his diabetes, his obesity, his cholesterol disorder, and his high blood pressure.

1. Diabetes

I discussed my five pillar approach with George. I recommended my diet, exercise, vitamins, and stress management treatment. Of course, the fifth pillar—prescription medications—was also vital to his renewed health.

Initially I kept George on the same dose of insulin and added Glucophage 500 mg twice a day. Unfortunately, Glucophage had to be stopped because he developed nausea and abdominal discomfort. In place of Glucophage, I added Precose 25 mg three times a day. At that time, Actos and Avandia were not yet available.

At five months, George's fasting blood glucose was 185 mg/dl, indicating that his diabetes was still uncontrolled. At that time, Rezulin, the first TZD drug, had just become available in the U.S. I placed him on Rezulin 600 mg/day. (Actos and Avandia, the other TZD drugs, became available two years later.)

At eight months, control of diabetes had improved remarkably, with a fasting blood glucose of 133 mg/dl. His HbA1c had come down to 7.5%.

At ten months, George's fasting blood glucose was even better with a value of 109 mg/dl. At this point, I added Glucotrol XL 20 mg/day and stopped his insulin shots. He was thrilled to be off insulin injections.

At twenty-two months, I again tried George on Glucophage. This time he tolerated it well. I gradually increased the dose of Glucophage to 1000 mg twice a day.

At thirty-five months, I switched George's Rezulin to Actos 45 mg/day, as Rezulin was withdrawn from the U.S. market due to its association with some cases of liver toxicity. (George had no liver problems on Rezulin.)

At forty months, George's HbA1c was 7.5% indicating fairly good control of diabetes. His HbA1c has continued to improve and has stayed under 6.5% in the last three years.

2. Cholesterol Disorder

With better control of his insulin resistance, George's triglyceride level came down and HDL (good) cholesterol went up, although still not in the optimal range.

CHOLESTEROL CONTROL

	Baseline	5 Months	10 Months	40 Months
Triglycerides	962 mg/dl	430 mg/dl	338 mg/dl	368 mg/dl
HDL Cholesterol	22 mg/dl	23 mg/dl	23 mg/dl	31 mg/dl
LDL Cholesterol	N/A*	N/A*	78 mg/dl	41 mg/dl

* LDL cholesterol could not be calculated due to high triglyceride level.

I switched George from Zocor to Lipitor 40 mg twice a day for insurance reasons. Both of these are statin drugs and each one is very effective in lowering LDL (bad) cholesterol.

3. High Blood Pressure

To treat his high blood pressure, I initially kept George on Vasotec 15 mg twice a day and Procardia XL 60 mg/day.

At eight months, I increased Vasotec to 20 mg twice a day (maximum dose).

At twenty-eight months, I switched Vasotec to Accupril 40 mg/day and gradually increased it to 40 mg twice a day, but still I could not get his blood pressure into the desired range of less than 130/80 mm Hg. At that point, I added Atacand 32 mg/day, and finally his blood pressure came into the target range.

BLOOD PRESSURE CONTROL

	Baseline	8 Months	10 Months	28 Months	40 Months
Blood Pressure	148/70 mm Hg	160/80 mm Hg	140/70 mm Hg	140/70 mm Hg	130/60 mm Hg

Accupril is a more tissue-specific ACE inhibitor. In my opinion, it is a better ACE inhibitor than Vasotec.

Atacand is a new drug for blood pressure control and belongs to a new class of blood pressure lowering drugs known as angiotensin receptor blocking drugs (ARBs for short).

At forty months, George underwent another coronary angiogram. His cardiologist was pleasantly surprised to find that his coronary artery disease had significantly improved.

George has been under my care for nine years and has not required any more angioplasties. Prior to my treatment, George had three angioplasties in only two years despite standard medical treatment. Only after I treated his diabetes with a focus on insulin resistance did his cycle of repeated angioplasties halt. His latest angiogram documented the effectiveness of my treatment approach. The disease process in his coronary arteries not only halted, but the condition of his blood vessels actually improved.

Risk for a Heart Attack Even After Bypass Surgery

An acute heart event, such as chest pain, brings patients to the hospital and to the likely diagnosis of a narrowing of the coronary arteries. Usually, they undergo angioplasty, stent placement, and /or heart bypass surgery. These procedures are only temporary solutions to relieve an acute emergency situation and don't treat the underlying cause of the problem: Insulin Resistance Syndrome.

Unfortunately, even at this stage, most patients are not diagnosed with Insulin Resistance Syndrome. Patients think their problem is fixed and they'll be fine as long as they eat right and take their drugs to lower cholesterol.

As demonstrated above, the process of Insulin Resistance Syndrome and, consequently, narrowing of the blood vessels continues until one day they are again rushed back to the hospital with chest pain only to find they are having another heart attack. Even after heart bypass surgery, it's essential to treat the real cause of narrowing of the coronary arteries—Insulin Resistance Syndrome.

o   o   o

Martin, a fifty-six-year old Caucasian male, had a history of high blood pressure for several years. One day he started having shoulder and jaw pain and was rushed to the ER. Martin was diagnosed with a heart attack. He underwent emergency angioplasty and, three days later, quadruple bypass surgery. At that time, he was also diagnosed with Type 2 diabetes. Following the conventional protocol, his physician treated his diabetes with glyburide.

After his discharge from the hospital, Martin became very active in the cardiac rehabilitation exercise program. He also followed his diet closely under the supervision of a dietitian. In three months, he lost about 40 lbs and started having low blood sugar. At that point, his physician took him off glyburide.

Six months later, he came to see me for a second opinion as one of his friends had told him about my new approach to treating diabetes and heart disease.

Medications

Lipitor 10 mg/day, Toprol Xl 100 mg/day, vitamin E 400 IU/day
Vitamin C 500 mg twice a day, aspirin 1/day

Physical Examination

Blood pressure = 120/70 mm Hg
Weight = 197 lbs (about 10 lbs overweight)

Laboratory Results

Fasting blood glucose = 117 mg/dl (should be 70–100 mg/dl)
Hemoglobin A1c = 5.9 % (should be less than 6.0%)
Triglycerides = 198 mg/dl (should be less than 150 mg/dl)
HDL cholesterol = 35 mg/dl (should be more than 40mg/dl in males)
LDL cholesterol = 71 mg/dl (should be less than 100 mg/dl in diabetics)
Total cholesterol = 146 mg/dl

Diagnosis

Even though Martin's LDL cholesterol was nicely controlled with Lipitor, and he had good control of his blood glucose through his diet and exercise, his HDL cholesterol was still too low and his triglyceride level was too high. This indicated that his insulin resistance was not under good control. I diagnosed him with Insulin Resistance Syndrome.

Treatment

I advised Martin to go on Rezulin in order to effectively reduce his insulin resistance, but he refused as he did not want to take one more pill, especially one that was a new drug. (At that time, Actos and Avandia were not yet available.)

At two months, Martin's triglycerides rose to 255 mg/dl. His HDL cholesterol further dropped down to 32 mg/dl.

His blood pressure was 170/80 mm Hg, so I placed him on Accupril 10 mg/day. I again advised him to take Rezulin. Once again, he refused because it was a new drug, but he did agree to take Glucophage instead, as it had been on the U.S. market for a few years.

At five months, Martin was evaluated by his cardiologist and underwent a treadmill exercise test, which he failed. His cardiologist did another angiogram, which showed that his grafts from his bypass surgery had already occluded (closed up). An angioplasty was performed and he was sent home.

Martin was understandably demoralized to learn that his grafts occluded after only two years despite his religious adherence to diet, exercise, and excellent control of blood glucose. Finally, he was willing to change course and adopt my treatment plan.

Martin and I discussed a plan to take charge of his diabetes—the five pillar plan. In addition to my diet, vitamin, and stress management plan, as well as his continued exercise, I started him on Rezulin 400 mg/day.

At seven months, Martin's HDL cholesterol went up to 45 mg/dl. His triglyceride level came down to 87 mg/dl. His LDL cholesterol was 59 mg/dl. His blood pressure was 130/70 mm Hg. His fasting blood glucose was 119 mg/dl.

At twelve months, I switched Martin from Rezulin to Actos 30 mg/day because Rezulin was withdrawn from the U.S. market due to its association with liver toxicity in some individuals. Martin, however, did not have any liver problems.

At fourteen months, Martin's HDL went up to 53 mg/dl. His triglyceride level came down to 54 mg/dl. His fasting blood glucose was 123 mg/dl. His hemoglobin A1c was 5.5%.

At that time, Martin's cardiologist performed another treadmill exercise test, and this time he passed with flying colors.

At thirty months from his initial consultation with me, also the most recent visit, he continues to do well. No chest pain, no angioplasties. He goes to the gym on a regular basis. His most recent lab test results were as follows:

HDL cholesterol = 56 mg/dl

Triglycerides = 91 mg/dl

LDL cholesterol = 51 mg/dl

Hemoglobin A1c = 5.6%

Fasting blood glucose = 117 mg/dl

Recently, Martin underwent another treadmill exercise test, which he again passed with flying colors.

For many diabetic patients like Martin, heart bypass surgery is a temporary fix. Again, like most patients in this medical scenario, Martin wasn't treated for his Insulin Resistance Syndrome. He was just placed on a cholesterol lowering drug that did its job of lowering his LDL (bad) cholesterol, but his HDL (good) cholesterol remained low and triglycerides remained high, indicating ongoing insulin resistance.

At the time of his heart bypass surgery, Martin was diagnosed with Type 2 diabetes, another manifestation of insulin resistance. Unfortunately, his insulin resistance was still neither diagnosed nor treated. Instead, he was treated with glyburide, the conventional way of treating blood glucose without any regard to insulin resistance.

To me, it's no surprise he developed narrowing of the grafts to his heart two years after heart bypass surgery. Now that his insulin resistance is under control, it's no surprise that he no longer experiences heart problems.

Stroke in Diabetics

A person suffers a stroke when blood flow is cut off from an area of the brain. This results in a neurological symptom, depending on the area of the brain involved.

The usual symptoms of a stroke include weakness in the leg, arm, or an entire side of the body. Sometimes, one side of the face is affected, causing slurred speech, difficulty in swallowing, and deviation of the angle of the mouth to one side. Sometimes, a stroke may cause blurry vision, imbalance, confusion, and even lack of consciousness. About 50% of stroke survivors live with permanent disabilities such as difficulty in walking, impaired speech, difficulty in self-care, and memory loss. Many stroke survivors visit the hospital numerous times with all sorts of medical problems including frequent pneumonias, recurrent strokes, heart attacks, and bedsores. Most become depressed. Their families also experience physical, emotional, and economic turmoil. Prevention of stroke is the key to this huge medical and psychosocial problem.

Stroke is the third leading cause of death in the United States. The general assumption that stroke is a disease of old age is not a reliable nor an accurate view. A lot of people under the age of

sixty-five have strokes. The incidence of stroke more than dou-
bles for each decade after the age of fifty-five.

There are three types of strokes:

- Ischemic strokes
- Embolic strokes
- Hemorrhagic strokes

Ischemic strokes are the most common. These strokes take
place when a blood clot forms in an already narrowed blood vessel of the brain. A transient ischemic attack, or TIA, is a minor
ischemic stroke.

An embolic stroke occurs when a blood clot forms inside the
heart, dislodges, travels to the brain, and blocks a small blood
vessel there.

A hemorrhagic stroke occurs when there is bleeding inside the
brain.

Risk for a Stroke

You are at risk for a stroke if you have any of the following risk
factors. The more risk factors you have, the higher the risk of
having a stroke.

- Diabetes
- Older than forty-five years old
- Overweight, especially around the waistline. This is also
  called abdominal obesity (waistline more than 35 inches in
  women and more than 38 inches in men; among Asians, these
  numbers are 32 inches for women and 35 inches for men).
- High blood pressure (more than 130/85 mm Hg)

- Low HDL cholesterol (less than 50 mg/dl in females; less than 40 mg/dl in males)
- High triglycerides (more than 150 mg/dl)
- Smoking
- Atrial fibrillation (irregular heart beat)
- Family history of stroke

These risk factors usually don't cause any symptoms. A stroke or a heart attack is usually the first symptom.

People want to ignore these risk factors as long as they feel fine. They don't understand that by the time they have symptoms, the quality of their life may never be the same.

Most diabetic patients have abdominal obesity, high level of triglycerides, low levels of HDL (good) cholesterol, and high blood pressure. All of these metabolic disorders are major risk factors for a stroke. Again, collectively, these disorders are known as Insulin Resistance Syndrome.

In my practice, I often see middle-aged diabetic patients with high blood pressure. When I tell them they have high blood pressure and need drug therapy, they look surprised and question my diagnosis of hypertension. Sometimes they say, "But my other physician didn't say any thing about it" or "Last month I had it checked at the free screening at the pharmacy and they said it was fine." My favorite line is, "My blood pressure is high because I'm in your office."

Accepting the diagnosis of diabetes, high blood pressure, and cholesterol disorder means that your body is no longer perfect and you must do something about it. Some people take the ostrich approach. They stick their head in the sand and hope it goes away. It's easier to be in denial than to face reality. Diabetes, high blood pressure, and cholesterol disorder need your attention. Don't ignore them.

Strokes are preventable. Early diagnosis and aggressive treatment of the risk factors is the key to the prevention of a stroke. In most diabetic patients, a stroke occurs due to narrowing of the blood vessels in the neck and/or in the brain.

Strategies to prevent a stroke in a diabetic are the same as in preventing a heart attack, discussed earlier in this chapter.

Memory Loss/Dementia in Diabetics

Dementia means a progressive decline in intellectual functioning. Memory loss is a frequent symptom of dementia.

Narrowing of the brain vessels is the underlying cause for intellectual decline and memory loss in a majority of diabetic patients. Transient ischemic attacks (TIAs), also known as ministrokes, take place due to transient cessation of blood circulation to a certain part of the brain. Multiple ministrokes over a period of time lead to the death of brain cells and, eventually, a person starts experiencing a decline in intellectual function and lapses in memory. This is known as multi-infarct dementia or vascular dementia, the most common cause for memory loss in diabetic patients.

Of course, the underlying cause for narrowing of the blood vessels is Insulin Resistance Syndrome. And once again, diabetes, high blood pressure, cholesterol disorder, and abdominal obesity are the main components of Insulin Resistance Syndrome.

In a recent, large clinical study involving 10,963 people, changes in cognitive function were assessed over a six-year interval.[1] Diabetes and hypertension were found to be the strongest predictors of decline in intellectual functioning, even as early as at the age of forty-seven.

In another study, researchers looked at the impact of ingesting 50 g of rapidly absorbing carbohydrates (one half of a bagel and white grape juice) on the memory of diabetic patients.[2] They found a positive correlation between carbohydrate intake and poor memory in these patients. In addition, overall poor control of diabetes was associated with a decline in memory.

If you don't aggressively treat the underlying disease that caused a stroke in the first place, how can you prevent further strokes and their consequences, such as memory loss? Quite often, these patients are misdiagnosed with Alzheimer's disease.

Another common problem is when patients suffer a heart attack, undergo heart bypass surgery or angioplasty, and they are not properly evaluated or treated for the risk factors for stroke. Remember, if you have narrowing of the blood vessels in your heart, you probably also have narrowing of the blood vessels in your brain.

Anyone who has memory loss, a stroke (even a minor stroke), a heart attack, coronary angioplasty, or heart bypass surgery should be evaluated for risk factors for narrowing of the blood vessels. These risk factors include hypertension, cholesterol disorder, and diabetes or prediabetes.

Other Causes of Memory Loss/Dementia

Besides vascular dementia, some of the other causes for memory loss or dementia include an underactive thyroid, vitamin B12 deficiency, subdural hematoma, AIDS, and syphilis. Out of these causes, an underactive thyroid and vitamin B12 deficiency are the most common disorders. Both can be easily diagnosed with blood testing.

A low level of vitamin B12 is common in elderly diabetic individuals who are also on metformin. Vitamin B12 deficiency should be treated either with vitamin B12 injections or with vitamin B12 pills. (See chapter 8 for more on vitamin B12 deficiency.)

Alzheimer's dementia is a diagnosis of exclusion. That is, once all the treatable causes of dementia as mentioned above have been excluded, only then should a diagnosis of Alzheimer's be made.

Diagnostic Testing for Memory Loss/Dementia

- Two-hour oral glucose tolerance test to diagnose prediabetes or diabetes
- Cholesterol panel, which should include HDL, LDL, and triglycerides
- Ultrasound of carotid arteries to rule out narrowing of the neck arteries
- MRI of the brain to rule out any evidence of a recent or an old stroke
- A thyroid blood panel to diagnose an underactive thyroid
- A blood test for vitamin B12, syphilis, and AIDS

o   o   o

Robert, a seventy-three-year-old Asian male, was referred to me by his neurologist after he evaluated Robert for gradual memory loss. His diagnostic workup included an MRI of his brain that showed evidence of several small strokes in the past.

His neurologist appropriately ordered a two-hour oral glucose tolerance test that showed:

Fasting blood glucose 118 mg/dl (mildly elevated)

One-hour blood glucose 218 mg/dl

Two-hour blood glucose 241 mg/dl (more than 200 mg/dl is diagnostic for diabetes)

This confirmed that Robert indeed was a diabetic. His diabetes would have remained undiagnosed if he hadn't taken the two-hour oral glucose tolerance test.

Robert also had some numbness of his toes for some time, which is another complication of diabetes.

Robert's mother had diabetes. His brother had high blood pressure and had suffered a stroke.

Medications

Prevacid (for his gastroesophageal reflux disease)

Physical Examination

Blood pressure = 140/90 mm Hg
Weight = 179 lbs (about 20 lbs overweight)

Laboratory Results

Triglycerides = 115 mg/dl (should be less than 150 mg/dl)
HDL (good) cholesterol = 57 mg/dl (should be more than 40 mg/dl in males)
LDL (bad) cholesterol = 120 mg/dl (should be less than 100 mg/dl in diabetics)

Diagnosis

I diagnosed Robert with Insulin Resistance Syndrome as he had Type 2 diabetes and high blood pressure. I concluded that he had developed narrowing of his brain arteries as a complication of Insulin Resistance Syndrome and, consequently, suffered several small strokes which led to memory loss.

Treatment

I educated him about diabetes and Insulin Resistance Syndrome. I treated him with my five pillar approach. I advised him about diet, exercise, and stress management and placed him on Glupride Multi and Actos 15 mg/day.

Initially Robert lost about 30 lbs, but then gradually gained about 10 lbs back. Now he is maintaining his weight at around 160 lbs.

Over the last two years Robert has done very well. His diabetes is under excellent control. His triglycerides came down by treating his underlying insulin resistance. His LDL cholesterol also came down with diet alone. His blood pressure has stayed in the 100–120/60–70 mm Hg range without any blood pressure medications. He has not had any more strokes. His memory and intellectual functioning is good for his age. The numbness in his toes is much improved.

DIABETES CONTROL

	Baseline	4 Months	12 Months	24 Months	27 Months
Fasting Blood Glucose	118 mg/dl	96 mg/dl	98 mg/dl	102 mg/dl	97 mg/dl
HbA1c	6.3%	6.0 %	5.7 %	5.9 %	5.8%

CHOLESTEROL CONTROL

	Baseline	4 Months	12 Months	18 months
Triglycerides	115 mg/dl	50 mg/dl	58 mg/dl	82 mg/dl
HDL Cholesterol	57 mg/dl	49 mg/dl	61 mg/dl	52 mg/dl
LDL Cholesterol	120 mg/dl	93 mg/dl	72 mg/dl	104 mg/dl

Kidney Disease in Diabetics

In the U.S., diabetes is one of the major reasons why patients develop kidney failure. The other major reason is high blood pressure. According to recent estimates by the National Institute of Health, diabetes is the single largest cause of kidney failure in the U.S. accounting for approximately 40% of all cases. These patients then require chronic dialysis or a kidney transplant to stay alive.

It's estimated that kidney failure requiring dialysis will develop in 20% to 40% of Type 2 diabetics who have diabetes for more than ten years. By the year 2020, it's estimated that 80% of dialysis patients will be Type 2 diabetics.

Diabetes, along with high blood pressure, affects kidney function slowly over a period of years. You don't develop symptoms due to diabetic kidney disease until it is too late and you're about to go on dialysis. Remember, diabetes is a silent killer.

Often people have the misconception that if you're urinating fine, then your kidney must be functioning normally. Wrong! You will continue to urinate without symptoms while diabetes and high blood pressure damage your kidneys. Pain, burning, or difficulty urinating are usually symptoms of urinary bladder infection or prostate enlargement, not kidney disease.

People often mistakenly think that pain in the lumber region is due to kidney disease. Pain in the lumbar region is almost always due to diseases of the lumbar spine, such as a herniated disc, arthritis, or a muscle spasm. Only rarely are kidneys responsible for pain in the lumber region.

Another misconception is that if your kidney ultrasound or CT scan is normal, then your kidneys must be normal, too. The fact is that these imaging tests focus on structural problems in the kidneys, such as stone formation, obstruction, or tumors. Diabetes and high blood pressure, on the other hand, cause a slow decline in kidney function.

Diabetic kidney disease is diagnosed by utilizing blood and urine tests.

Before I discuss how diabetes affects your kidneys, let me first briefly explain what are the normal functions of the kidneys.

Normal Functions of the Kidneys

By far, the most important function of the kidneys is to form urine and, thereby, remove waste products of cellular metabolism from the blood stream and deposit them into the urine.

The basic functioning unit of the kidneys is called the nephron. The formation of urine takes place in the nephron as a result of filtration of water, electrolytes (such as sodium, potassium, and calcium), and waste products of the metabolism (such as creatinine from the muscles).

Clinically, the filtration rate of the kidneys is measured as creatinine clearance, a test that involves collecting urine for a twenty-four-hour period.

Blood urea nitrogen (BUN) and serum creatinine are the typical tests for kidney function and are included in most blood chemistry panels. Serum creatinine is a more accurate test for kidney function than BUN.

The other important functions of the kidneys include:

- Regulation of electrolytes (such as potassium, sodium, and calcium) in the blood
- Maintaining adequate hydration
- Regulation of blood pressure
- Regulation of vitamin D metabolism
- Production of a hormone, erythropoietin, which is important for the normal production of red blood cells

Stages in the Development of Diabetic Kidney Disease

Diabetes affects kidneys slowly over a period of years and causes a progressive decrease in kidney functions. We divide this gradual decline in kidney functions into five stages.

Stage 1: Hyperfiltration

There is an increase in the filtration rate at the nephron level, which is the basic functioning unit of the kidney.

Normal creatinine clearance is 80–120 ml/minute. In the stage of hyperfiltration, the creatinine clearance rate may be as high as 170 ml/minute or more. In the blood chemistry panel, BUN and creatinine are normal at this stage.

Patients do not have any symptoms at this stage of diabetic kidney disease, which usually lasts several years.

Diabetic kidney disease is easily halted and even reversed at this point. Therefore, it is very important to diagnose kidney disease at this stage. This can easily be accomplished by measuring creatinine clearance, which requires a twenty-four-hour urine collection.

Stage 2: Microalbuminuria

At this stage, albumin, a special protein, starts to leak into the urine due to damage to the wall of the nephron. Clinically, this albumin leakage can be detected by measuring albumin excretion in the urine. A urinary albumin excretion of more than 30 mg but less than 300 mg in a twenty-four-hour period is known as microalbuminuria. In the blood chemistry panel, BUN and creatinine are usually normal at this stage.

As with Stage 1 diabetic kidney disease, patients do not have any symptoms of diabetic kidney disease at this stage, which usually lasts for several years.

Routine urine testing does not detect this small amount of albumin excretion. Instead, three special methods of screening for microalbumin excretion are available:

- Twenty-four-hour urine collection
- Measurement of albumin-to-creatinine ratio in a random spot collection
- Timed (four hours or overnight) urine collection

Diabetic kidney disease at this stage can be halted and even reversed in a majority of patients.

Diabetics with microalbuminuria should be treated with an ACE inhibitor or an angiotensin receptor blocking drug (ARB), provided there are no contraindications and even if their blood pressure is not elevated. See page 199 for more details on ACE inhibitors and angiotensin receptor blocking drugs.

Stage 3: Frank Proteinuria

With further progression of diabetic kidney disease, larger quantities of albumin start to spill into the urine. If a twenty-four-hour urine albumin excretion exceeds 300 mg in twenty-four hours, it is called frank proteinuria. In the blood chemistry panel, BUN and creatinine may be abnormal at this stage. This stage of diabetic kidney disease may last a few years.

Patients in this stage may start experiencing some ankle swelling. Many patients, however, do not experience any symptoms at this stage.

Until recently, most patients in this stage used to have a poor prognosis, ultimately requiring dialysis in a few years. However, with the combination of new antidiabetic drugs such as Actos (pioglitazone) or Avandia (rosiglitazone) as well as ACE inhibitors and angiotensin receptor blocking drugs (ARBs), many patients in this stage can now halt further progression of kidney damage.

See page 199 for more details on ACE inhibitors and angiotensin receptor blocking drugs (ARBs).

Stage 4: Nephrotic Syndrome

With further progression of diabetic kidney disease, urinary protein excretion may reach several thousand milligrams per day. A proteinuria of more than 3000 mg in twenty-four hours is known as nephrotic range proteinuria. In the blood chemistry panel, BUN and creatinine are usually abnormal at this stage. Often patients have high blood pressure as well.

Patients with nephrotic syndrome usually have symptoms of leg swelling, abdominal swelling, and even shortness of breath, due to the accumulation of fluid inside the chest cavity.

Patients in this stage should be treated with aggressive control of diabetes, use of ACE inhibitors and/or angiotensin receptor blocking drugs and diuretics as needed.

Stage 5: End Stage Renal Disease

In this stage, patients have many symptoms such as fatigue, leg swelling, poor appetite, intractable itching, and mental confusion. In the blood chemistry panel, BUN and creatinine are always abnormal at this stage. Patients also have high blood pressure, which is usually difficult to treat.

These patients are treated with chronic dialysis, usually three times a week. They are prone to all sorts of complications, such as infections and clotting of the dialysis access, low blood counts, high risk for bleeding, vitamin D deficiency, parathyroid disease, and osteoporosis. These patients are also at a very high risk for heart attacks, strokes, and leg amputations. They are usually frequent visitors to the hospital. Quality of life is often poor at this stage.

Preventing Kidney Disease

Fortunately, diabetic kidney disease can be prevented, but only with early diagnosis and aggressive treatment of diabetes and high blood pressure. Unfortunately, diabetes and hypertension remain undiagnosed and untreated in millions of people worldwide. By the time diabetes is diagnosed, a number of people have already developed diabetic kidney disease.

Several excellent clinical studies have demonstrated that aggressive control of blood glucose and high blood pressure can significantly reduce the risk for kidney failure.

By using the five pillar treatment approach, I have been able to prevent end stage renal disease in the vast majority of my diabetic patients.

Recommendations to Prevent Kidney Failure in Diabetics

1. Good Control of Diabetes

Kidney disease primarily develops in those patients who have poor control of diabetes. Excellent control of diabetes can prevent development of kidney disease. I set the following targets for controlling diabetes in my patients.

Target Blood Glucose Values

- Premeal blood glucose levels should be 70–120 mg/dl, preferably less than 100 mg/dl
- Two-hour postmeal blood glucose levels should be less than 140 mg/dl, preferably less than 120 mg/dl
- Hemoglobin A1c (HbA1c) should be less than 6.0%

2. Good Control of Blood Pressure

Hypertension should be aggressively treated in diabetic patients. I aim for blood pressure to be less than 120/80 mm Hg in most of my diabetic patients.

The selection of drugs to control blood pressure is important. I use angiotensin converting enzyme inhibitors (ACE inhibitors) or angiotensin receptor blocking drugs (ARBs) as the first choice for drugs that treat high blood pressure in diabetic patients. Several excellent scientific studies have clearly demonstrated that ACE inhibitors as well as ARBs not only control high blood pressure, but also preserve kidney function.

Other drugs that can be used to treat severe high blood pressure include:

- Diuretics, in small doses (such as hydrochlorthiazide or indapamide)
- Calcium channel blockers (such as Norvasc, diltiazem, or verapamil)
- Alpha blockers (such as Cardura)
- Beta-blockers (such as atenolol or metoprolol)
- Centrally acting drugs such as clonidine

3. Urinary Albumin Excretion and Creatinine Clearance Test

This special urine test should be done on a yearly basis. A routine urine test does not check for it. This yearly testing should start at the time of diagnosis in Type 2 diabetic patients. In Type 1 diabetic patients, yearly measurements should be started five years after the diagnosis of diabetes.

4. Use of an ACE Inhibitor or ARB Drug

Diabetic patients who have microalbuminuria should be given an ACE inhibitor or an angiotensin receptor blocking (ARB) drug even if their blood pressure is not elevated.

A number of well-designed scientific studies have shown that ACE inhibitors as well as ARBs (angiotensin receptor blocking) can reduce microalbuminuria and preserve kidney function in diabetic patients.

Commonly Used ACE Inhibitors in the U.S.

Brand Name	Generic Name
Altace	Ramipril
Accupril	Quinapril
Aceon	Perindopril
Lotensin	Benazepril
Monopril	Fosinopril
Zestril/Prinivil	Lisinopril
Vasotec	Enalapril
Capoten	Captopril

Commonly Used Angiotensin Receptor Blocking Drugs (ARBs) in the U.S.

Brand Name	Generic Name
Diovan	Valsartan
Cozaar	Losartan
Avapro	Irbesartan
Atacand	Candesartan
Micardis	Telmisartan
Benicar	Olmesartan

5. Management of Cholesterol

Cholesterol disorder, which is almost always present in patients with Type 2 diabetes, must be treated aggressively.

Target Cholesterol Levels
- LDL cholesterol should be less than 100 mg/dl
- HDL cholesterol should be greater than 50 mg/dl
- Triglyceride level should be less than 100 mg/dl

o   o   o

Mark, a forty-four-year-old Caucasian male, was diagnosed with diabetes at the time of his angioplasty for his heart attack. His fasting blood glucose was in the 200–329 mg/dl range during his hospital stay. Mark also had a history of cholesterol problems.

He was sent home on Glucotrol and Plavix and was advised to seek an endocrine consultation. He came to see me one month after his hospital discharge.

His mother and two brothers had diabetes.

Medications

Glucotrol XL 10 mg/day, Plavix 75 mg/day

Physical Examination

Blood Pressure = 130/80 mm Hg
Weight = 170 lbs (25 lbs overweight)
Abdominal obesity was present

Diagnosis

Mark had microalbuminuria, which indicated early kidney disease due to diabetes. In addition to diabetes, he also had low HDL, high triglycerides and abdominal obesity, which are other

LABORATORY RESULTS

Test	Result	
Twenty-four-hour Urinary Albumin Excretion	61 mg in twenty-four hours	Should be less than 30 mg in twenty-four hours
Fasting Blood Glucose	122 mg/dl	Should be less than 100 mg/dl
Hemoglobin A1c	7.2%	Should be less than 6.0%
Triglycerides	192 mg/dl	Should be less than 150 mg/dl, preferably less than 100 mg/dl
HDL Cholesterol	27 mg/dl	In males, should be more than 40 mg/dl, preferably more than 50 mg/dl
LDL Cholesterol	172 mg/dl	Should be less than 100 mg/dl in diabetics

components of Insulin Resistance Syndrome. His LDL cholesterol was also high. He developed coronary heart disease primarily due to Insulin Resistance Syndrome and high LDL cholesterol.

Treatment

I discussed my five pillar approach including diet, exercise, vitamins, stress management, and drugs.

1. Kidney Disease

I placed Mark on an ACE-inhibitor, Monopril 10 mg/day, to treat his microalbuminuria.

At three months, I switched Monopril to Accupril 10 mg/day (Accupril is a more tissue specific ACE-inhibitor than Monopril).

At seven months, I increased the dose of Accupril to 20 mg/day.

At fifteen months, Mark's microalbuminuria had almost normalized.

KIDNEY CONTROL

	Baseline	15 Months
Microalbumin Excretion in Twenty-four Hours	61 mg	37 mg

2. Diabetes

I stopped his Glucotrol, as I did not want to stimulate his pancreas to produce more insulin since his problem was insulin resistance and not insulin production.

Instead, I started him on Glucophage 500 mg three times a day and Rezulin 400 mg/day. Later, I switched his Rezulin to Actos because Rezulin was taken off the U.S. market due to its association with liver toxicity.

With my five pillar treatment strategy, I was able to achieve excellent control of his blood glucose as evidenced by his hemoglobin A1c coming down from 7.2% at the start of treatment to 5.9% at fifteen months.

DIABETES CONTROL

	Baseline	11 Months	15 Months
Fasting Blood Glucose	122 mg/dl	100 mg/dl	101 mg/dl
Hemoglobin A1c	7.2%	6.2%	5.9%

4. Blood pressure

Monopril and, subsequently, Accupril kept Mark's blood pressure below 120/80 mm Hg, which is the desirable level in patients with diabetic kidney disease.

BLOOD PRESSURE CONTROL

	Baseline	3 Months	7 Months	11 Months	15 Months
Blood Pressure	130/80 mm Hg	105/60 mm Hg	100/60 mm Hg	120/70 mm Hg	110/60 mm Hg

5. Cholesterol Disorder

I started Mark on Lipitor 10 mg/day to control his cholesterol disorder. At three months, his LDL cholesterol was within target level. With improvement in insulin resistance, his triglycerides reached the target level. His HDL cholesterol was improving, although still not in the optimal range.

CHOLESTEROL CONTROL

	Baseline	3 Months	11 Months
Triglycerides	192 mg/dl	91 mg/dl	96 mg/dl
HDL Cholesterol	27 mg/dl	29 mg/dl	32 mg/dl
LDL Cholesterol	172 mg/dl	61 mg/dl	67 mg/dl

Nerve Disease in Diabetics

Nerve disease in diabetic patients can take different forms.

- Diabetes usually affects peripheral nerves in the feet, legs, and at times, the hands; this is known as peripheral neuropathy
- Diabetes also frequently affects the autonomic nervous system, giving rise to autonomic neuropathy

Diabetic Peripheral Neuropathy

Diabetic peripheral neuropathy usually causes symptoms such as tingling, a pins-and-needles sensation, a burning sensation, numbness, or pain. Initially, it affects the toes, which progresses to the entire foot and eventually can progress to the entire lower leg. Later in the course of the disease, hands can also be involved. Symptoms are usually worse at night and can interfere with sleep.

The diagnosis of peripheral neuropathy is often missed. According to the results of an excellent study reported at the 63rd Scientific Sessions of the American Diabetes Association in 2003, physicians failed to diagnose peripheral neuropathy in 62% of patients.

Numb feet are at a high risk for injury, such as by accidental scalding from hot water or by accidental puncture, like a small piece of gravel into the sole of the foot. Because of a lack of sensation, wounds go unnoticed, especially in between the toes and on the soles of the feet. Infection settles in these wounds and can cause serious destruction to soft tissues and even extend to the underlying bone. Bone infection is very difficult to treat and may require amputation and a prolonged course of antibiotics.

Early diagnosis is important in order to prevent further progression of this complication. An endocrinologist and a neurologist can diagnose peripheral neuropathy at an early stage. Often it requires specialized diagnostic testing.

Peripheral neuropathy often starts years before a person is diagnosed with diabetes. An oral glucose tolerance test (OGTT) can diagnose diabetes as well as prediabetes many years earlier. See chapter 2, Diagnosis of Diabetes, for further details on early diagnosis.

Other factors that can contribute toward peripheral neuropathy:

- Vitamin B12 deficiency, which is common in those on metformin
- Excessive alcohol use
- Vitamin D, calcium, potassium, and magnesium deficiencies often mimic symptoms of peripheral neuropathy. Vitamin D deficiency is commonly present in elderly patients as well as

in individuals who avoid sun exposure. Potassium and magnesium deficiencies are frequently present in patients who are on diuretics.

Prevention Is the Best Treatment

Tight blood glucose control can prevent the development of peripheral neuropathy. Therefore, excellent blood glucose control is crucial right from the time of the diagnosis of diabetes.

Treatment Options for Peripheral Neuropathy

Again, good control of diabetes using my five pillar treatment strategy is crucial, as it prevents further progression of neuropathy.

A spouse or a friend should regularly examine your feet for any ulcer or sign of infection.

See a podiatrist on a regular basis.

There are also some vitamin therapies and prescription medications that can help reduce the symptoms of peripheral neuropathy.

1. Alpha-Lipoic Acid. As discussed in chapter 8, alpha-lipoic acid is a dietary supplement that has been used in Germany for more than thirty years for the treatment of diabetic neuropathy. In Germany, fifteen clinical trials have been completed that have shown the effectiveness of alpha-lipoic acid in treating peripheral neuropathy. Currently, clinical trials are under way in the U.S.

I use alpha-lipoic acid in my diabetic patients with peripheral neuropathy and have seen some good results. I feel that this product is safe. I have not seen any serious side effects in my patients. The usual dose is 600–1200 mg/day.

2. Capsaicin. For superficial, burning-type pain, capsaicin works pretty well. It is a skin cream that is applied to the affected area, usually the feet. Capsaicin is derived from hot red peppers. It takes about two to three weeks before the pain starts subsiding. Beware! Initially it may cause some worsening of pain.

3. *Cymbalta (Duloxetine).* In 2004, the drug Cymbalta was approved for the treatment of diabetic peripheral neuropathy. It works well in about 60% of patients. Most common side effects include dry mouth, nausea, constipation, diarrhea, dizziness, and hot flashes.

4. *Neurontin (Gabapentin).* Neurontin is an antiseizure drug that is often used to treat the pain of peripheral neuropathy. Most patients tolerate this drug fairly well. Drowsiness, dizziness, and fatigue are the typical complaints I have heard from patients who are on this medication, especially at higher doses.

On rare occasions, other seizure medications such as Dilantin (phenytoin) and Tegretol (carbamazepine) are used to treat diabetic peripheral neuropathy. These drugs have serious side effects and should only be prescribed by a physician knowledgeable about these drugs.

5. *Nortriptyline, Amitriptyline, Desipramine.* These are older antidepression drugs that have been used to treat the pain of peripheral neuropathy. Patients often do not tolerate these drugs well due to their common side effects, which include drowsiness, dizziness, dry mouth, impotence, retention of urine, and heart arrhythmias. These drugs *must not* be used in patients with a history of glaucoma, urinary retention, and heart arrhythmias.

6. *Mexitil (Mexiletine).* Mexitil is a heart medicine used to treat arrhythmia. It has also been used to treat diabetic peripheral neuropathy. Due to its potential serious side effects, this drug should

only be prescribed by a physician experienced in prescribing this drug, such as a cardiologist.

o   o   o

Steve, a thirty-seven-year-old Caucasian male, developed symptoms of excruciating pain in his feet, excessive urination, and excessive thirst about six months prior to seeing me. After testing, he was found to have a markedly elevated blood glucose level of 294 mg/dl and was diagnosed with diabetes. His primary care physician started him on Glucovance 1.25/250 a day (Glucovance is a combination of glyburide and metformin). His doctor referred him to me for further management.

Physical Examination

Blood pressure = 135/95 mm Hg
Weight = 206 lbs (about 25 lbs overweight)

Laboratory Results

Fasting blood glucose = 273 mg/dl (should be less than 100 mg/dl)
Hemoglobin A1c = 11.7% (should be less than 6.0%)
Triglycerides = 150 mg/dl (should be less than 150 mg/dl)
HDL cholesterol = 34 mg/dl (should be more than 40 mg/dl in males)
LDL cholesterol = 127 mg/dl (should be less than 100 mg/dl in diabetics)

Diagnosis

I diagnosed Steve with Insulin Resistance Syndrome consisting of diabetes, high blood pressure, and low HDL cholesterol. I suspected that the pain in his feet was due to diabetic peripheral neuropathy. I also referred Steve to a neurologist for further diagnostic testing and treatment of his peripheral neuropathy.

Treatment

Steve and I discussed my five pillar approach, including diet, exercise, vitamins, stress management, and drugs.

1. Diabetes

Using my treatment triangle approach, I placed him on Actos 45 mg/day and continued Glucovance. Within two months, his diabetes came under excellent control.

At six months, I switched Glucovance to Glucophage 1000 mg twice a day. Steve has maintained excellent control of his diabetes over the four years he has been under my care.

DIABETES CONTROL

	Baseline	2 Months	12 Months	25 Months	36 Months	45 Months
Fasting Blood Glucose	273 mg/dl	98 mg/dl	109 mg/dl	98 mg/dl	97 mg/dl	102 mg/dl
Hemoglobin A1cC	11.7%	5.9%	5.6%	5.2%	5.2%	5.1%

2. Peripheral Neuropathy

Steve was started on Neurontin 300 mg/day, which was gradually increased over several months to 600 mg four times a day to control his disabling pain. It took many months before his excruciating pain started to improve. Later, I added alpha-lipoic acid, which helped to bring the dose of Neurontin down to 600 mg two times a day. On this regimen, his pain of neuropathy is under good control.

At four years after his initial diagnosis, his neurologist repeated his nerve conduction study and was truly amazed to find out that not only did Steve's neuropathy not worsen (as is the usual course), but it had also markedly improved. This reversal of diabetic peripheral neuropathy is unheard of in medical literature. For me, nothing is more rewarding than to see results like this in my patients. Steve is very pleased with the progress he has made.

3. Hypertension

A prescription for Altace 2.5 mg/day has nicely controlled Steve's high blood pressure over these last four years.

Diabetic Autonomic Neuropathy

The autonomic nervous system controls the function of our various organs such as the heart, stomach, intestine, urinary bladder, and, in men, the penis. Diabetes often affects this autonomic nervous system and can cause the following symptoms:

- Fullness and bloating in the upper abdomen after eating. This happens due to the slowing of stomach emptying. Technically, this condition is known as diabetic gastroparesis.
- Chronic diarrhea
- Chronic constipation
- Impotence
- Urinary incontinence
- Dizziness upon standing due to a drop in blood pressure
- Excessive sweating
- Heart arrhythmia (excessively fast or slow heart rate)

Physicians often forget to think of diabetic autonomic neuropathy as a cause of these symptoms. As a result, patients usually undergo an extensive diagnostic workup that does not accurately diagnose their problem. Patients often undergo procedures such as CT scans, MRI scans, colonoscopies, and gastroscopies. These procedures might detect anatomic problems, but autonomic neuropathy affects the function of an organ, and, therefore, does not show up on these tests.

An experienced endocrinologist is your best bet in diagnosing these disorders correctly. Most of these disorders are diagnosed clinically and require the clinical skills of an endocrinologist.

Some specialized tests are used to confirm the clinical diagnosis of autonomic dysfunction. A special test that involves a test meal can accurately assess the emptying of the stomach and, therefore, diagnose diabetic gastroparesis. Autonomic neuropathy of the heart can be diagnosed with a test known as the heart rate variability test.

Treatment of Diabetic Autonomic Neuropathy

Good control of diabetes can prevent further progression of the problems associated with diabetic autonomic neuropathy. Therefore, aim for excellent control of diabetes, targeting your hemoglobin A1c to be less than 6.0%.

Each of these conditions should be properly diagnosed by an experienced physician and treated accordingly.

o   o   o

Edward, a seventy-nine-year-old Caucasian male, was referred by his family physician for the management of thyroid cancer. His thyroid cancer had been treated with surgery and radiation six years ago. He was in remission with a good long-term prognosis.

Edward had been experiencing numbness of his feet, excessive urination, and impotence for some time. Review of his medical records from his family physician's office showed that his fasting blood level was elevated as 123 mg/dl two months ago. Edward said he was unaware that his fasting blood sugar level was elevated.

Edward had been diagnosed with high blood pressure and had also undergone a heart pacemaker placement three months before he came to me.

Medications

Zestril 20 mg twice a day
Terazosin 2 mg/day
Vitamin D 50,000 units/day
Calcium citrate 4 tablets/day
Synthroid 200 mcg/day

Physical Examination

Blood pressure = 150/100 mm Hg
Weight = 208 lbs (about 25 lbs overweight)

Diagnosis

I repeated Edward's fasting blood glucose test which turned out to be 155 mg/dl, confirming the diagnosis of diabetes. I assessed the numbness in his feet to be due to diabetic peripheral neuropathy. I assessed that his impotence was due to diabetic autonomic neuropathy. The heart pacemaker was placed to treat his arrhythmia, another manifestation of autonomic neuropathy.

Treatment

I explained my five pillar approach to him, discussing diet, exercise, vitamins, stress management, and drugs. I placed him on Actos 15 mg/day. After three months, he was feeling much better. The numbness in his feet as well as his fatigue were improving. His diabetes had come under excellent control as evidenced by his HgA1c decreasing from 7.0% to 5.7% in just three months of treatment.

Edward has continued to maintain excellent control of his diabetes over the last six years that he has been under my care. Numbness in his feet due to peripheral neuropathy is much improved. Though it has not significantly improved, his impotence has not worsened. He has not developed any other manifestations of diabetic autonomic neuropathy.

Impotence in Diabetics

Impotence is common among diabetics. However, impotence can be due to a variety of reasons other than diabetes and, therefore, should be thoroughly evaluated by an expert in this field, preferably an endocrinologist.

Various causes of impotence include:

- Autonomic neuropathy due to uncontrolled diabetes
- Poor circulation due to diabetes and Insulin Resistance Syndrome
- Smoking
- Excessive alcohol consumption
- Certain drugs such as beta-blockers, thiazide diuretics, spironolactone, clonidine, antidepressants, antianxiety drugs, cimetidine, ranitidine, metoclopramide, and soy products
- Low testosterone level
- High prolactin level, a hormone produced by the pituitary gland
- Prostate surgery
- Psychological problems

In most diabetic patients, impotence is a complex problem. There are multiple factors working in concert that lead to impotence.

- Usually, diabetes is uncontrolled
- The patient is not on insulin-sensitizing drugs, which are Actos, Avandia, and metformin
- The patient is on beta-blockers to control hypertension
- HDL cholesterol is low and triglycerides are high
- Circulation is poor
- The patient feels quite tired all the time due to a variety of reasons including uncontrolled diabetes, obesity, side effects of medicines, lack of vitamin D and other vitamins and minerals, and the stress of daily life. You are not interested in sex when you're tired, fatigued, and stressed out.
- Often these patients are depressed; having sex is the last thing on their mind

Treatment of Impotence

Treatment of impotence is quite challenging. My approach to the treatment of impotence in diabetic patients is as follows:

- First, I thoroughly evaluate a patient for all of the causes mentioned above
- I treat all the factors that I can identify in an individual patient
- I treat their diabetes as well as other components of Insulin Resistance Syndrome, such as hypertension and cholesterol disorder, aggressively with my new treatment approach
- I try to stop any medicines that may contribute to impotence, such as beta-blockers, spironolactone, metoclopramide, or soy products

- I make sure prolactin is not elevated and testosterone levels are normal for the patient's age
- I strongly encourage smokers to quit smoking
- Those who are overweight are encouraged to lose weight, which also helps increase energy
- With proper amounts of vitamin D, calcium, potassium, magnesium, and other mineral supplements, they start feeling better
- I also address their depression with my stress management strategy
- After correcting all of these factors, I sometimes prescribe drugs such as Viagra, Cialis, or Levitra

Viagra

Viagra must be taken about an hour before sexual activity. Headache, flushing, and dizziness are frequent complaints that I have heard from my patients using Viagra.

Please note that Viagra use has caused several deaths. Therefore, you should be very careful about using this drug. Patients on nitrates and alpha blockers such as Cardura (doxazosin), Hytrin (terazosin) must not use Viagra. Patients with heart disease should check with their cardiologist before using Viagra.

Cialis and Levitra

After Viagra, two other drugs called Cialis and Levitra were released in the U.S. for treatment of impotence. These are in the same class of drugs as Viagra. Their onset of action is faster than Viagra. Cialis is effective during a twenty-four-hour period after its intake. Therefore, you have more flexibility about the timing of your sexual activity. Side effects of both Cialis and Levitra are similar to side effects of Viagra.

Other Options

Other older treatment options for impotence include a vacuum pump, injection of Caverject into the penis, MUSE, and lastly, a penile implant.

A *vacuum pump* works for some patients. Patients taking blood thinners should avoid it. A vacuum pump may cause bruising of the penis.

With *Caverject* a special chemical known as prostaglandin E1 is delivered by injection into the penis. You need to learn the injection technique from a nurse at a urologist's office. Penile pain and excessive stimulation of the penis are the main problems with these injections. However, it works in most people with impotence.

With *MUSE (Medicated Urethral System for Erection)*, prostaglandin E1 is delivered through the opening at the tip of the penis. Penile pain, excessive stimulation of the penis, and dizziness are the main problems with this technique. It works in about 50% of patients with impotence.

A *penile implant* should be the last resort. It involves surgery that has its own complications.

Poor Circulation in the Legs

Diabetics frequently have poor circulation in their legs, which can eventually lead to amputation. The typical symptom of poor circulation is pain in the legs, especially while walking, that subsides upon resting. In severe cases, this pain is present even at rest.

Poor circulation develops due to narrowing of the arterial blood vessels, a complication of Insulin Resistance Syndrome. Narrowing of blood vessels is a generalized process affecting all arterial blood vessels in the body. If you have blockages of the coronary arteries in your heart, you may also have blockages in the arterial blood vessels in your legs, brain, and intestines. I often see patients who have undergone angioplasty of their heart arteries but are totally unaware that they may also have poor circulation in their legs.

Diagnostic Testing for Poor Circulation in the Legs

You should have a Doppler ultrasound test of your leg arteries if you have symptoms of poor circulation. This is a simple, noninvasive, outpatient test that can easily diagnose peripheral arterial disease in the legs.

In most patients, treatment is with medications and no further testing is required. In patients with severe peripheral arterial disease, angioplasty or surgery is sometimes required. In these patients, an angiogram of the leg arteries is done prior to an angioplasty or surgery.

Treatment

Prevention is the best treatment. Early diagnosis and appropriate treatment of diabetes can prevent this devastating complication of diabetes. With my five pillar treatment approach to diabetes, I have been able to prevent leg amputation in the vast majority of my patients.

Once you've developed poor circulation in your legs, aggressive control of diabetes and other components of Insulin Resistance Syndrome with appropriate drugs can prevent further progression of this disease and may save your limbs.

Patients who smoke cigarettes are putting fuel on the fire. Smokers *must* quit smoking in order to prevent leg amputation.

Certain drugs such as Trental (pentoxifylline) and Pletal (cilostazol) may help in the treatment of poor circulation.

Eye Disease in Diabetics

Diabetes gradually affects eyes over a period of years. It affects the innermost layer of the eye, known as the retina. Hence, the condition is known as diabetic retinopathy.

Diabetes is the leading cause of blindness in the U.S. Fortunately, this debilitating condition can be prevented by aggressive treatment of diabetes right from the start. In a landmark study, DCCT (Diabetes Control and Complication Trial), the risk for diabetic retinopathy was decreased by 76% with tight control of blood glucose.[3] At the Jamila Diabetes & Endocrine Medical Center, I have been able to prevent diabetic retinopathy in the vast majority of my patients.

Current recommendations to prevent diabetic eye disease are:

1. Yearly Eye Examination

Diabetics should see an optometrist /ophthalmologist on a yearly basis to diagnosis eye disease at an early stage. This annual eye examination should start at the time of diagnosis for Type 2 diabetics. Type 1 diabetics should have yearly eye examinations starting five years after the diagnosis of diabetes.

2. Aggressive Control of Blood Glucose in Most Diabetic Patients

Target blood glucose values:

- Before meal blood glucose should be 70–120 mg/dl, preferably less than 100 mg/dl
- Two-hour after-meal blood glucose should be less than 140 mg/dl, preferably less than 120 mg/dl
- Hemoglobin A1c (HbA1c) should be less than 6.0%

3. Aggressive Control of High Blood Pressure

Blood pressure should be less than 120/80 mm Hg in a diabetic patient. Any blood pressure value above 130/80 mm Hg is high and is called hypertension. It should be aggressively treated.

Hypertension occurs much more frequently in patients with diabetes. Hypertension itself can cause eye damage. Therefore, the combination of hypertension and diabetes is very detrimental for eyes.

Fatty Liver in Diabetics

Uncontrolled diabetes can also affect your liver. This condition is known as fatty liver, which simply means increased deposition of fat in your liver. This condition can affect the functioning of your liver, which is detected on blood tests. Often, you don't have any symptoms due to this condition. However, in some cases it can lead to cirrhosis of the liver, which is a very serious disease that is often fatal.

Diagnosis of Fatty Liver

ALT (alanine aminotransferase), AST (aspartate aminotransferase), bilirubin, and albumin are blood tests for liver function and are included in most blood chemistry panels. Elevation in ALT and AST is usually the first indication of liver disease including fatty liver.

The most common causes for abnormal liver function include fatty liver, drugs, alcoholism, and hepatitis. Your physician needs to carefully look into these common causes for abnormal liver function.

In a nonalcoholic, diabetic person, if the hepatitis risk panel is negative and you are not taking a drug causing liver toxicity, then fatty liver is the likely diagnosis.

o   o   o

Joseph, a fifty-eight-year-old Caucasian, consulted me for his diabetes. About one year prior, he experienced fatigue and weight loss. He was diagnosed with diabetes as his fasting blood glucose was elevated at 416 mg/dl; in addition, his triglycerides were elevated at 208 mg/dl, HDL cholesterol was 48 mg/dl, and LDL cholesterol was 143 mg/dl. At the time of his diagnosis, he decided to control his diabetes with diet and exercise alone. He denied any alcohol abuse.

His father and paternal grandmother also had Type 2 diabetes. One brother had high blood pressure and both of his brothers had coronary heart disease.

Medications

None

Physical Examination

Blood Pressure = 130/90 mm Hg
Weight = 186 lbs
Height = 5'5"
(about 40 lbs overweight)

Laboratory Results

Fasting blood glucose = 154 mg/dl (should be less than 100 mg/dl)

HbA1c = 8.3% (should be less than 6.0%)

Triglycerides = 204 mg/dl (should be less than 150 mg/dl)

HDL Cholesterol = 40 mg/dl (should be more than 40 mg/dl in males)

LDL Cholesterol = 134 mg/dl (should be less than 100 mg/dl in diabetics)

ALT = 67 u/l (should be less than 45 u/l)

His bilirubin and albumin were normal.

Diagnosis

I diagnosed Joseph with Insulin Resistance Syndrome, consisting of abdominal obesity, Type 2 diabetes, elevated triglycerides, and relatively low HDL cholesterol. He was not an alcoholic and was not on any medicines. Also, he did not have any risk factors for hepatitis. I suspected his elevated ALT was due to fatty liver.

Treatment

I gave him my recommendations on diet, exercise, vitamins, stress management, and drugs. I placed him on Glupride Multi, Actos 45 mg/day, Glucophage 500 mg daily at dinner time, and

Zocor 20 mg/day. With this treatment strategy, his diabetes and cholesterol disorder came under excellent control.

Within one month, his ALT nicely came down to a near normal level of 48 u/l. At four months, his ALT completely normalized and has stayed normal.

ALT (Liver Function Test)

	Baseline	1 Month	4 Months	6 Months	9 Months
ALT	67 u/l	48 u/l	41 u/l	33 u/l	32 u/l

DIABETES CONTROL

	Baseline	1 Month	2 Months	4 Months	13 Months	15 Months
Fasting Blood Glucose	154 mg/dl	142 mg/dl	117 mg/dl	112 mg/dl	135 mg/dl	144 mg/dl
Hemoglobin A1c	8.3%		6.4%	6.2%	6.5%	6.1%

CHOLESTEROL CONTROL

	Baseline	2 Months	9 Months	15 Months
HDL Cholesterol	40 mg/dl	57 mg/dl	59 mg/dl	65 mg/dl
Triglycerides	204 mg/dl	176 mg/dl	137 mg/dl	129 mg/dl
LDL Cholesterol	134 mg/dl	108 mg/dl	115 mg/dl	105 mg/dl

Decreased Immunity Against Infections

If your diabetes is uncontrolled, your immune system can't fight off infections effectively. High blood glucose itself weakens your immune system. In addition, uncontrolled diabetes frequently leads to poor circulation, especially in the legs. Because of poor circulation, your immune cells have difficulty reaching an infected area of the skin. That is why a skin wound, which would easily heal in a nondiabetic, may become a nonhealing wound in a diabetic. Sometimes, the end result is an amputation of the toe, foot, or even leg.

Helpful Tips for Avoiding Infections

- Take good care of your diabetes. Aim for good control of your blood glucose while being careful to avoid hypoglycemia. Good control of blood glucose helps to improve your immune function. Please refer to chapter 12 for guidelines about monitoring your diabetes.
- Stress wreaks havoc on our immune system. Stress management should become part of your daily routine. Please refer to chapter 7 for information about stress management.
- Take commonsense precautions to avoid infections. For example, never walk barefoot. This may prevent a small, dirty, sharp object from puncturing the bottom of your foot. This small precaution may end up saving your leg.
- Take any infection seriously. Notify your doctor promptly and seek advice.

Diabetic Ketoacidosis

Diabetic ketoacidosis is a life-threatening complication of diabetes. Typically, Type 1 diabetics are more prone to it, but it does rarely occur in Type 2 diabetics as well. An initial episode of diabetic ketoacidosis is the first manifestation of diabetes in some Type 1 diabetics.

In this condition, there is a lack of insulin, which results in a rapid rise in blood glucose accompanied by an increase in special chemicals in the body known as ketone bodies. Blood PH changes from neutral to acidic, hence the term ketoacidosis.

If you have ketoacidosis, your breath becomes rapid, shallow, and has a fruity smell to it. You may experience nausea, vomiting, and even abdominal pain. Severe fatigue develops and, if untreated, you could lapse into a coma and even die.

Causes of Diabetic Ketoacidosis

Usually an infection is the precipitating factor for diabetic ketoacidosis. Often the site of infection is obvious, but sometimes the infection is not visible. Skin infection in the form of an abscess is a common culprit.

A common scenario is that a Type 1 diabetic develops nausea or vomiting from an acute stomach illness, such as the flu. Since they're unable to eat, they think they shouldn't take insulin. Unfortunately, sometimes diabetics get this erroneous, disastrous advice from a health care professional! This is a perfect setup for the development of diabetic ketoacidosis.

Diabetics on insulin pumps are at special risk for diabetic ketoacidosis due to several factors. Abscess development at the needle site can push you into diabetic ketoacidosis. Lack of insulin from an empty insulin reservoir, mechanical failure of the pump, or kinks in the tubing can lead to the development of diabetic ketoacidosis.

Sometimes the stress of a medical illness such as an acute heart attack, a stroke, or an acute abdominal illness may throw you into diabetic ketoacidosis. More often what happens is that in the hospital emergency room, in the midst of the hoopla of an acute heart attack or a stroke or some other acute medical illness, no one thinks to give you insulin while you're waiting hours for the results of diagnostic testing.

Another case scenario is when you become unconscious, for example, in a traffic accident, and no one taking care of you realizes that you are a Type 1 diabetic on insulin. You don't receive insulin and lapse into diabetic ketoacidosis.

For all these reasons, if you're a diabetic on insulin, it's essential that you wear a bracelet carrying your medical information.

Diabetic ketoacidosis is a true medical emergency and must be treated in a hospital setting under the supervision of a knowledgeable physician.

Coma in Diabetics

A diabetic patient is at a high risk for a coma. In addition to typical causes for comas, such as a head injury or brain infection, diabetics are at risk for special types of comas:

- Hypoglycemic coma
- Diabetic ketoacidosis (DKA) coma
- Hyperglycemic hyperosmolar nonketotic (HHN) coma

Please refer to chapter 12 for more information on hypoglycemia.

Hyperglycemic hyperosmolar nonketotic (HHN) coma is mainly seen in elderly diabetic patients, although it can occur at any age. It develops gradually and occurs due to severely uncontrolled diabetes and dehydration. In the days before losing consciousness, a patient complains of excessive thirst, frequent urination, and extreme fatigue. Sometimes it is precipitated by a high dose of steroid therapy, an acute illness such as pneumonia, or an acute heart attack.

Treatment must be carried out in a hospital setting under the supervision of a knowledgeable physician. Mortality rate is high, as much as 50%.

CHAPTER 12

Monitoring Guidelines

In order to assess the effectiveness of your treatment strategy, you need to monitor certain parameters. Only then will you be able to monitor your progress (or lack of progress) and make appropriate adjustments to your treatment plan.

In this chapter, I explain the guidelines I give my patients to monitor their progress. In most diabetic patients, our goal is:

- To achieve good control of blood glucose level
- To minimize the risk of low blood glucose (hypoglycemia)
- To keep blood pressure in the normal range
- To detect cholesterol disorder and keep it under control
- To watch for any signs of diabetes effecting the kidneys, eyes, or feet

Monitoring of Blood Glucose

Target Blood Glucose Values

I tell my patients to aim for the following values for their blood glucose.

- Premeal blood glucose should be 70–120 mg/dl, preferably less than 100 mg/dl
- Two-hour after-meal blood glucose should be less than 140 mg/dl, preferably less than 120mg/dl

Frequency of Blood Glucose Testing

If you are a Type 2 diabetic, you should test your blood glucose about two hours after each meal. However, after a while, this does become cumbersome. Pricking your fingers several times a day is no fun. I tell my patients to rotate the timing of testing each day. For example, one day check it two hours after breakfast, the next day two hours after lunch, and the third day do it two hours after dinner.

The two-hour after-meal blood glucose value is particularly important for the following reasons. The two-hour after-meal blood glucose is closely linked to the risk for heart attack. It shows the impact of your food on your blood glucose. The two-hour after-meal blood glucose value should be less than 140 mg/dl, preferably less than 120 mg/dl. A value of more than 140 mg/dl indicates that you either ate too much or you ate the wrong food or a combination of these two factors. You should write down what you eat. Soon you will know what to eat and what to avoid. Share this diary with your doctor on each visit.

If you are a Type 1 diabetic, then ideally you should check your blood glucose six times a day: before each meal and two hours after each meal. You check your blood glucose before each meal to calculate the dose of short-acting insulin that you need. The rationale for two-hour after-meal glucose is to see the impact of that particular meal on your blood glucose and also to see if you took enough short-acting insulin to cover that meal.

Other Tips for Type 1 and Type 2

- Check your blood glucose whenever you are weak, dizzy, or confused
- Record all of these blood glucose values, along with your meal and any symptoms in a log
- Do *not* forget to bring your log to your appointment with your physician. New glucose meters have the ability to store blood glucose values in their memory.

Hemoglobin A1c (HbA1c)

Hemoglobin A1c (HbA1c) is a blood test that measures overall blood glucose values around the clock for the preceding three months. Therefore, it should be checked every three months.

At the Jamila Diabetes & Endocrine Medical Center, the target goal for my diabetic patients is an HbA1c of less than 6%. A significant number of patients have been able to achieve this goal. A few even have an HgA1c of less than 5.5%. Patients with an HbA1c of less than 6% rarely suffer from the complications of diabetes.

Seventy-two-hour Continuous Glucose Monitoring

If your diabetes is way out of control or there are wide fluctuations in your blood glucose levels, you may ask your physician to order a seventy-two-hour continuous glucose monitor test. In this test, you wear a device about the size of a cell phone hooked to a plastic catheter that has a plastic needle at the end. This needle is inserted under your skin by a physician. This device checks your glucose every hour for seventy-two hours (three days and three nights) and can pinpoint the cause of wide fluctuations in your glucose levels. Then your physician can make appropriate adjustments in your medications.

At the Jamila Diabetes & Endocrine Medical Center, I find this test to be extremely useful in difficult cases of diabetes where the cause for wide fluctuations in glucose levels is not apparent or when a patient's diabetes is severely uncontrolled.

Factors that Can Affect Blood Glucose Values

Diet

If you eat a meal that is high in carbohydrates, your blood glucose will go high and it may take a while before you return to normal blood glucose values. For details on diet, please refer to chapter 6.

Exercise

In Type 2 diabetics, exercise typically lowers blood glucose. Therefore, it's a good idea to go for a walk after a meal.

However, in some Type 1 diabetics, exercise may initially cause an increase in blood glucose and then a sudden drop. Therefore, Type 1 diabetics should check their blood glucose before exercise. If it is more than 250 mg/dl, then wait for about an hour. Check it again and make sure it's coming down before you start to exercise. If pre-exercise blood glucose is less than 100 mg/dl, then eat a small snack before exercising.

For more details on exercise, please refer to chapter 7.

Stress

Both physical and mental stresses can cause an increase in blood glucose.

For more details on stress, please refer to chapter 7.

Menses

Typically, menses can increase your blood glucose. So, monitor your blood glucose more frequently during your menstrual period and adjust the dose of insulin (or insulin stimulating drugs) accordingly.

Medications

Certain medications can influence your blood glucose. The common ones are:

1. Steroids. Typically, for arthritis, tendonitis, asthma, or a skin disorder, a specialist may treat your condition with a steroid. Many cancer chemotherapy protocols also include steroids. You receive steroids in the form of an injection or pills. Subsequently, you experience a rise in your blood glucose. You wonder what is raising your blood glucose, especially if your specialist did not warn you that your diabetes will get out of control with the addition of steroids.

Knowledge of the connection between steroids and a rise in blood glucose can prepare you to deal with your blood glucose escalating after steroid treatments. You should check your blood glucose more frequently after such treatment and make adjustments in the dose of your diabetes medications in consultation with your endocrinologist.

2. Beta-Blockers. These drugs are typically used in patients with hypertension and heart disease. Common beta-blockers include: atenolol, propranolol, metoprolol, and sotalol.

These drugs can worsen insulin resistance and therefore should be used with caution in patients with Type 2 diabetes and insulin resistance.

Beta-blocker drugs can also complicate hypoglycemia. The body responds to hypoglycemia by producing catecholamines that cause symptoms of hypoglycemia, such as sweating and heart pounding. Beta-blocker drugs interfere with the actions of catecholamines and, therefore, can interfere with the symptoms of hypoglycemia. In other words, you may have hypoglycemia and not be aware of it. So beware and discuss this issue with your physician to make sure that the potential benefits of a beta-blocker drug outweigh its potential risks.

3. *Birth Control Pills/Hormone Replacement Therapy.* Birth control pills as well as hormone replacement therapy in menopausal women may worsen insulin resistance, which can increase your blood glucose values. So watch your blood glucose closely if you decide to go on birth control pills or hormone replacement therapy.

Hospitalization

I often find my diabetic patients with good control of their diabetes go to the hospital for some acute illness and discover that their diabetes has now soared out of control. Everyone wonders what happened.

A number of factors are usually responsible for this phenomenon.

- Stress (physical and mental) of the acute illness. Imagine being in the busy ER of a hospital while you wait several hours before someone sees you.
- Intravenous fluids. Almost everyone ends up receiving them while in the hospital. Often they contain glucose.
- Diet. Patients typically receive a diet high in calories as well as high in carbohydrates.

• Interruption of antidiabetic drugs. Often patients do not receive their antidiabetic drugs while waiting to be seen, waiting for their tests results, or waiting for admission.

Low Blood Glucose and How to Treat It

Educate yourself as well as your family members about low blood glucose, technically known as hypoglycemia. If your blood glucose goes below 70 mg/dl, you have low blood glucose. The lower the blood glucose, the more severe your hypoglycemia will be.

Most people have minimal symptoms at blood glucose levels between 70–60 mg/dl, moderate symptoms at levels between 60–40 mg/dl, and will pass out if their blood glucose is below 40 mg/dl.

Symptoms of Hypoglycemia

The usual initial symptoms of mild to moderate hypoglycemia are:

• Heart pounding
• Cold sweats
• Dizziness
• Weakness
• Abdominal discomfort

Symptoms of more severe hypoglycemia include:

• Headache
• Foggy thinking
• Blurred vision
• Disorientation

- Feeling of passing out
- Seizure
- Coma

You need to understand that the above mentioned symptoms are not specific to hypoglycemia alone. These symptoms may be due to other medical conditions as well.

For example, cold sweats, pounding of the heart, and a feeling of passing out are also symptoms of a heart attack. As a diabetic, you are also at a high risk for a heart attack.

Foggy thinking, disorientation, headache, and blurred vision may be due to a stroke or migraine headache. Being a diabetic places you at high risk for a stroke.

These symptoms may also be due to a very high blood glucose level.

Drugs that Can Cause Hypoglycemia

- Insulin
- Sulfonylurea drugs, including Glucotrol (glipizide), Micronase (glyburide), Diabeta (glyburide), Glynase (glyburide), Amaryl (glimepiride), and Diabinese (chlorpropamide)
- Starlix (nateglinide)and Prandin (repaglinide)
- Precose

Drugs that *Do Not* Cause Hypoglycemia

These drugs do not cause hypoglycemia by themselves, but in combination with the above mentioned drugs, hypoglycemia can occur.

- Glucophage, Fortamet, Glumetza (metformin)
- Actos (pioglitazone)
- Avandia (rosiglitazone)

Treatment for Hypoglycemia

If you have symptoms of hypoglycemia, but do *not* have a feeling of passing out, then check your blood glucose level. If it is above 70 mg/dl, you do not have hypoglycemia. Your symptoms may be due to other reasons, such as a heart attack or stroke. Time to call 911.

If for some reason you cannot check your blood glucose and are on one of the drugs that can cause hypoglycemia, then presume you have hypoglycemia and ingest glucose in any form available, such as fruit juice, regular sugar, candy, or glucose tablets.

Note: hypoglycemia due to Precose does not respond to regular sugar but only to glucose tablets.

If you have blurry vision, disorientation, or a feeling of passing out but are conscious, then presume that you have hypoglycemia and drink some glucose in any available form.

Check your blood glucose in about fifteen minutes. Usually by that time, you should be feeling better and your blood glucose should be above 70 mg/dl. Then, you should also eat a snack or a meal (if it's meal time) and skip your diabetes medicine for that meal. Also call your doctor for further advice.

If you become unconscious, your spouse, friend, or companion should give you a glucagon shot and call 911. You should be taken to a nearby hospital and properly evaluated.

Hypoglycemia due to sulfonylurea drugs and long-acting insulin can recur within twenty-four hours. In patients with kidney failure, this dangerous period may last up to seventy-two hours as these drugs linger in the body for a much longer period. Hypoglycemia due to short-acting insulins such as Starlix, Prandin, and Precose can recur within a couple of hours.

Every patient on insulin should have a glucagon kit nearby in order to treat hypoglycemia. A family member, friend, or teacher should know about this glucagon kit and should give this injection to the patient in case he/she becomes unconscious. Glucagon acts rapidly to raise blood glucose and can save a patient's life.

If you had an episode of moderate to severe hypoglycemia, you should be monitored in a hospital.

Other Useful Tips about Hypoglycemia

- Type 1 diabetics are at a higher risk for hypoglycemia than Type 2 diabetics.
- Patients with kidney failure who are on insulin or oral hypoglycemic diabetic drugs are at a higher risk for hypoglycemia as compared to those without kidney failure.
- Some diabetic patients, especially Type 1 diabetics of long duration, can develop a situation where they become hypoglycemic without any symptoms. This is known as hypoglycemia unawareness and can be life-threatening. If you have this condition, you should be treated by an experienced endocrinologist.
- Nocturnal hypoglycemia (hypoglycemia at night) often develops because of short-acting insulin taken at bed time. This can be avoided by not taking any short acting insulin at bedtime. A protein snack at bedtime can also help prevent nocturnal hypoglycemia.
- Every diabetic patient, especially Type 1 diabetics, should wear a medic alert bracelet.

Monitoring Blood Pressure

In many diabetics, blood pressure is also high, which needs close monitoring and treatment as necessary. Target blood pressure in diabetics should be less than 130/80 mm Hg, preferably less than 120/80 mm Hg.

Any reduction in blood pressure reduces the risk of complications, with the lowest risk in those with a systolic blood pressure less than 115 mm Hg and diastolic blood pressure less than 75 mm Hg.

At the Jamila Diabetes & Endocrine Medical Center, I have been able to lower blood pressure to less than 130/80 mm Hg in a majority of my patients. A number of these patients have a blood pressure of less than 115/75 mm Hg. The risk for complications is markedly reduced in these patients.

Caution

Blood pressure readings are only as good as the equipment used as well as the person checking it. Many free or low-cost blood pressure kits targeted to patients may not give accurate readings. Even in a physician's office, blood pressure readings are dependent upon the equipment used as well as the technique of the person checking it. At the Jamila Diabetes & Endocrine Medical Center, I personally check blood pressure on each and every one of my patients.

Monitoring Cholesterol

In diabetics with Insulin Resistance Syndrome, there are unique cholesterol abnormalities. Typically, in Type 2 diabetics, HDL (good) cholesterol is low, triglyceride level is high, and LDL (bad) cholesterol is more harmful (Type B rather than Type A) as compared to nondiabetics.

LDL cholesterol is of two patterns: Type B and A. Type B cholesterol particles are small and dense. They are more easily deposited in the blood vessel wall as compared to Type A particles, which are large, fluffy, and buoyant. In Type 2 diabetics, the LDL cholesterol pattern is typically Type B. That is why cholesterol gets deposited in the blood vessels of diabetics more easily than nondiabetics.

Deposition of LDL cholesterol in the blood vessel wall causes inflammation of the vessel wall. This inflammation of the vessel wall can be easily detected by a blood test called a sensitive or cardio CRP (C-reactive protein).

HDL cholesterol is called good cholesterol because it cleanses out the cholesterol buildup in the blood vessel wall. There are also two types of HDL cholesterol: HDL 2 and HDL 3. HDL 2 cholesterol particles are large and buoyant and are the most protective. In most Type 2 diabetics, total HDL cholesterol and especially HDL 2 cholesterol is low.

It's important to pay attention to all the various subtypes of cholesterol, rather than just the total cholesterol. Many patients only want to know their total cholesterol number. They have the misconception that if their total cholesterol is less than 200 mg/dl, they're safe. Nothing can be further from the truth!

Target Cholesterol Levels

- Aim for total HDL cholesterol to be greater than 50 mg/dl, the higher the better (HDL 2 should be at least more than 10 mg/dl in males and more than 15 mg/dl in females)
- Aim for triglyceride levels of less than 100 mg/dl
- Aim for LDL cholesterol to be less than 100 mg/dl, preferably below 70 mg/dl

- Aim for LDL Type A
- Aim for sensitive or cardio CRP to be less than 1mg/l

At the Jamila Diabetes & Endocrine Medical Center, I have been able to achieve these target cholesterol levels in most of my diabetic patients.

Monitoring for Diabetic Kidney Disease

At the early stages of diabetic kidney disease, albumin, a special protein, starts to leak into the urine due to damage to the wall of the nephron, the basic unit of the kidneys. Clinically, this albumin leakage can be detected by measuring albumin excretion in the urine. This urinary albumin excretion testing should be done on a yearly basis starting at the time of diagnosis of diabetes in Type 2 diabetics and five years after the diagnosis of diabetes in Type 1 diabetics.

A urinary albumin excretion of more than 30 mg, but less than 300 mg in a twenty-four-hour period is known as microalbuminuria. Please note that routine urine testing does not detect this small amount of albumin excretion.

There are three special methods for detecting albumin excretion available:

- Twenty-four-hour urine collection
- Measurement of albumin-to-creatinine ratio in a random spot collection
- Timed (four hours or overnight) urine collection.

Diabetic kidney disease at this stage of microalbuminuria can be halted and even reversed in a majority of diabetic patients.

See chapter 11 on Kidney Disease in Diabetics for more details.

Monitoring for Diabetic Eye Disease

Diabetes can affect the innermost lining of the eye, known as the retina. Hence, the condition is called diabetic retinopathy.

A thorough eye examination, including retina examination, should be done by an ophthalmologist or an optometrist on a yearly basis, starting at the time of diagnosis for Type 2 diabetics. For Type 1 diabetics, this monitoring should start at five years after the diagnosis.

For details, please refer to chapter 11 on Eye Disease in Diabetics.

Monitoring of Feet

Diabetics are at high risk for numb or cold feet, which is often due to peripheral neuropathy and/or poor circulation in the legs. A small wound may develop unrecognized because there is no pain since the feet are numb due to neuropathy. These wounds easily become infected and set the stage for amputation. Therefore, a foot examination should be done for neuropathy (nerve disease), pulses, ulcers, fissures, calluses, and deformities at least once a year.

You should see a podiatrist to monitor your feet carefully on a regular basis. You, your spouse, or companion should also regularly examine your feet for any wounds. In case you see a wound, report it to your physician.

For more details, see chapter 11 on Diabetic Peripheral Neuropathy and Poor Circulation of the Legs.

NOTES

Chapter 2

1. Mokdad AH, Bowman BA, Ford ES, Vinicor F, Marks JS, Koplan JP. The continuing epidemic of obesity and diabetes in the United States. *JAMA* 2001; 286:1195–2000.

2. Ford ES. Insulin Resistance Syndrome: The public health challenge. *Endocr Pract* 2003; 9(suppl 2):23–25.

3. Hu FB, Leitzmann MF, Stampfer MJ, et al. Physical activity and television watching in relation to risk for type 2 diabetes mellitus in men. *Arch Intern Med* 2001; 161:1542–1548.

4. Manicardi V, Camellini L, Bellodi G, Coscelli C, Ferrannini E. Evidence for an association between high blood pressure and hyperinsulinemia in obese men. *J Clin Endocrinol Metabolism* 1986; 62(6):1302–4.

5. Pyorala K., Savolainen E, Kaukola S, Haapakoski J. Plasma insulin as coronary heart disease risk factor: relationship to other risk factors and predictive value during 9 1/2-year follow-up of the Helsinki Policemen Study. *Acta Med Scand Suppl* 1985; 701:38–52.

6. Eschwege E, Richard JL, Thibult N, et al. Coronary heart disease mortality in relation with diabetes, blood glucose and plasma insulin level. The Paris Prospective Study, ten years later. *Horm Metab Res Suppl* 1985; 15:41–46.

7. Moller LF, Jespersen J. Fasting serum insulin level and coronary heart disease in a Danish cohort: 17-year follow-up. *J Cardiovasc Risk* 1995; 2:235–240.

8. Despres J-P, Lamarche B, et al. Hyperinsulinemia as an independent risk factor for ischemic heart disease. *N Engl J Med* 1996; 334:952–957. Salomaa V, Riley W, Kaark JD, et al. Non–insulin dependent diabetes mellitus and fasting insulin concentrations are associated with arterial stiffness index, the ARIC study. *Circulation* 1995; 91:1432–1443.

9. Michels KB, Solomon CG, Hu FB, et al. Type 2 diabetes and subsequent incidence of breast cancer in the Nurses' Health Study. *Diabetes Care* 2003; 26:1752–1758.

10. Warram JH, Martin BC, Krolewski AS, et al. Slow glucose removal rate and hyperinsulinemia precede the development of type II diabetes in the offspring of diabetic parents. *Ann Intern Med*, 1990; 113:909–915.

11. Shimabukuro M, Zhou Y-T, LeviM, et al. Fatty acid–induced B-cell apoptosis: a link between obesity and diabetes. *Proc Natl Acad Sci USA* 1998; 95:2498–2502.

Chapter 3

1. Mokdad AH, Bowman BA, Ford ES, Vinicor F, Marks JS, Koplan JP. The continuing epidemic of obesity and diabetes in the United States. *JAMA* 2001; 286:1195–2000.

2. Rodriguez BL, Abbott RD, Fujimoto W, et al. The American Diabetes Association and World Health Organization classifications for diabetes. Their impact on diabetes prevalence and total and cardiovascular disease mortality in elderly Japanese-American men. *Diabetes Care* 2002; 25:951–955.

3. Tuomilehto J. A glucose tolerance test is important for clinical practice. *Diabetes Care* 2002; 25:1880–1882.

4. Lowe LP, Liu K, Greenland P, Metzger BE, Dyer AR, Stamler J.: Diabetes, asymptomatic hyperglycemia and 22-year mortality in black and white men: the Chicago Heart Association Detection Project in Industry Study. *Diabetes Care* 1997; 20:163–169.

5. Rodriguez BL, Lau N, Burchfiel CM, Abbott RD, Sharp DS, Yano K, Curb JD.: Glucose intolerance and 23-year risk of coronary heart disease and total mortality: the Honolulu Heart Program. *Diabetes Care* 1999; 22:1262–1265.

6. The Decode Study Group, on behalf of the European Diabetes Epidemiology Group. Glucose Tolerance and Cardiovascular Mortality. Comparison of fasting and 2-hour diagnostic criteria. *Arch Intern Med.* 2001; 161:397–404.

Chapter 6

1. United Kingdom Prospective Diabetes Study Group. Intensive blood-glucose control with sulphonylureas or insulin compared with conventional treatment and risk of complications in patients with type 2 diabetes (UKPDS 33). *Lancet.* 1998; 352:837–853.

Chapter 8

1. Evans JL, Goldfine ID. Alpha-lipoic acid: a multifunctional antioxidant that improves insulin sensitivity in patients with type 2 diabetes. *Diabetes Technol Ther 2000*; 2:401–413. Jacob S, Ruus P, Hermann R, et al. Oral administration of RAC-alpha-lipoic acid modulates insulin sensitivity in patients with type 2 diabetes mellitus: a placebo-controlled pilot trial. *Free Radic Biol Med* 1999; 27:309–314. Konrad T, Vicini P, Kusterer K, et al. Alpha-lipoic acid treatment decreases serum lactate and pyruvate concentrations and improves glucose effectiveness in lean and obese patients with type 2 diabetes. *Diabetes Care* 1999; 22:280–287. Ziegler D, Reljanovic M, Mehnert H, Gries FA. Alpha-lipoic acid in the treatment of diabetic polyneuropathy in Germany: current evidence from clinical trials. *Exp Clin Endocrinol Diabetes* 1999; 107:421–430.

2. Ziegler D, Reljanovic M, Mehnert H, Gries FA. Alpha-lipoic acid in the treatment of diabetic polyneuropathy in Germany: current evidence from clinical trials. *Exp Clin Endocrinol Diabetes* 1999; 107:421–430.

3. Richard Anderson, Nanzberg Cheng, Noella A, et al. Elevated intakes of supplemental Chromium improves glucose and insulin variables in individuals with Type 2 Diabetes. *Diabetes* 1997; 46:1786–1791.

4. Gupta A, Gupta R, Lal B. Effect of Trigonella foenum-graecum (fenugreek) seeds on glycaemic control and insulin resistance in Type 2 diabetes mellitus: a double blind placebo controlled study. *J Assoc Physicians India* 2001; 49:1057–1061.

5. Fratiac, Gordill BE, et al. Acute hypoglycemic effects of Opuntia streptacantha Lemmiare in NIDDM (Letter). *Diabetes Care* 1990; 13:455–256.

6. Khan A, Safdar M, Khan M, Khan N, Anderson R. Cinnamon improves glucose and lipids of people with type 2 diabetes. *Diabetes Care* 2003.

7. Rundek T, Naini A, Sacco R, Coates K, DiMauro S. Atorvastatin decreases the coenzyme Q10 level in the blood of patients at risk for cardiovascular disease and stroke. *Arch Neurol* 2004; 61:889–892.

8. Nadler, JL, Buchanan T, Natarajan R, et al. Magnesium deficiency produces insulin resistance and increased thromboxane synthesis. *Hypertension* 1993; 21:1024–1029.

Chapter 9

1. Koshiyama H, Shimono D, et al. Inhibitory effect of pioglitazone on carotid arterial wall thickness in type 2 diabetes. *J Clin Endocrinol Metab* 2001; 86(7):3452–6.

2. Yoshimoto T, Naruse M, et al. Vasculo-protective effects of insulin sensi-tizing agent pioglitazone in neointimal thickening and hypertensive vascular hypertrophy. *Atherosclerosis* 1999; 145(2):333–40.

3. Ovalle F, Bell DS. Clinical evidence of thiazolidinedione-induced improve-ment of pancreatic beta-cell function in patients with type 2 diabetes mellitus. *Diabetes Obes Metab* 2002; 4(1):56–9.

Chapter 11

1. Knopman D, et al. Atherosclerosis Risk in Communities (ARIC) cohort. *Neurology* 2001; 56:42–28.

2. Greenwood CE, Kaplan RJ, et al. Carbohydrate induced memory impair-ment in adults with type 2 diabetes. *Diabetes Care* 2003; 26:1961–1966.

3. The Diabetes Control and Complications Trial Research Group. The ef-fect of intensive treatment of diabetes on the development and progression of long term complications of insulin-dependent diabetes mellitus. *N Engl J Med* 1993; 329:977–986.

ACKNOWLEDGEMENTS

I gratefully acknowledge:

Jodie Rhodes, my literary agent, for believing in this project and working tirelessly with an unparalleled commitment.

Marnie Cochran, my editor, for her vision, insightful comments, and extraordinary patience.

Aqeel Zaidi, for coming up with the idea of the book. A true visionary.

Hasan Zaidi, for getting me on the road to become a doctor.

Waseem Zaidi, for living with diabetes, in a sensible and courageous way.

My father, for teaching me to speak the truth no matter what the consequences.

My mother, for showing me the path of wisdom, patience, and compassion.

INDEX